STREET SCENARIOS FOR THE EMT AND PARAMEDIC

Brent Braunworth
Albert L. Howe

Reviewed by Laurence W. Schlanger, M.D.

REGENTS/PRENTICE HALL, Upper Saddle River, New Jersey 07458

Editorial/production supervision,
    interior design, and page layout: *Barbara Marttine*
Cover design: *Yes Graphics*
Cover photo: *Linda Gheen*
Prepress buyer: *Ilene Sanford*
Manufacturing buyer: *Ed O'Dougherty*
Acquisitions editor: *Natalie Anderson*
Editorial assistant: *Wendy Rivers*

Printed in the United States of America

10   9   8

ISBN   089303-976-4

Prentice-Hall International (UK) Limited,London
Prentice-Hall of Australia Pty. Limited, Sydney
Prentice-Hall Canada Inc., Toronto
Prentice-Hall Hispanoamericana, S.A., Mexico
Prentice-Hall of India Private Limited, New Delhi
Prentice-Hall of Japan, Inc., Tokyo
Pearson Education Asia Pte. Ltd., Singapore
Editora Prentice-Hall do Brasil, Ltda., Rio de Janeiro

This book is dedicated to all those in EMS who have been awakened at 2 A.M. for a call in which the chief complaint is "pain behind the eyes during urination."

Thanks to Allyson and Mary, as well as our families and friends, for putting up with us throughout this whole ordeal.

Special thanks goes to those people who assisted in the photography segment by preparing, setting up, and appearing in the simulated scenarios.

CONTENTS

FOREWORD

Street Scenarios for the EMT and paramedic is designed to provide EMS personnel with a challenging set of practical problems for instruction and testing. Newly trained and experienced medical personnel continually encounter new ailments and emergencies or unfamiliar presentations of common problems. Even apparently simple and straightforward problems in emergency medicine can challenge the most experienced individuals. It would take a lifetime of encounters in medical practice to experience the vast spectrum of injury and disease. One way of telescoping the process is through case presentations among peers. We need not experience, personally, every disease in order to gain an understanding of it. Another method is the practical application of knowledge and techniques in predesigned scenarios using realistic situations, equipment, and actors masquerading as the ill or injured. In this way we can rehearse for what would otherwise be a perplexing and frightening situation if encountered for the first time in reality.

In medical school and residency training, hospitals and clinics provide the large numbers of patients the student must treat to gain indispensable experience. This is supplemented by the unending parade of case presentations and clinicopathologic conferences. Eventually, after several years of practice, the arrogant young physician will confide, "I have seen it all."

For EMTs and paramedics, the opportunity for hands-on experience is not as great. Many years can pass before the medic has had enough experience to feel comfortable managing the large variety of problems he or she may encounter. Our intention is that this book be used to bridge that gap between knowledge and experience. These scenarios can be used as a method of exposing the student to realistic situations and testing his or her ability to practically apply acquired knowledge.

Our intent is not to provide detailed explanations of specific therapies or pathophysiology, although you can use the scenarios as a springboard for a discussion of these entities. We have attempted to abide by nationally accepted criteria—Basic Cardiac Life Support, Basic Trauma Life Support, Prehospital Trauma Life Support, Advanced Trauma Life Support, Pediatric Advanced Life Support, and the new up-to-date Advanced Cardiac Life Support standards. We have also tried to avoid controversial methods of treatment. The latter is quite difficult since most current therapy is subject to controversy: the use of MAST; prophylactic lidocaine; the use of the esophageal airway; high-dose epinephrine; choices of IV fluid; even the value of the Trendelenburg position. Alas, medical therapy and treatment modalities, like fashions, come and go.

It is our hope that this book will increase the breadth of the student's experience in managing the common and the obscure, the simple and the complex cases; that it will be useful for training and testing EMTs and paramedics; and that it will stimulate discussion of all aspects of prehospital care and fundamental aspects of medicine.

We would like to thank the following reviewers who assisted in the development of this book:

Bryan E. Bledsoe, D.O., EMT-P, Emergency Physician, Baylor Medical Center, Waxahatchie, TX.

Kevin Crawford, Carlsbad Fire Department, Carlsbad, CA.

John K. Gaffney, BBA, NREMT-P 1/c, Center for Disaster Medicine, University of New Mexico, Albuquerque, NM.

Captain Lee Newsome, City of Ocala Fire Department, Ocala, FL.

Charly D. Miller, NREMT-P, Denver General Hospital, Denver, CO.

Robert Porter, M.A., EMT-P, Central New York EMS, Syracuse, N.Y.

Bruce Shade, NREMT-P, Commissioner of EMS, Cleveland, OH.

Todd M. Stanford, BS, PAC, MICD, Physicians Assistant, Emergency Department, United Hospital Center, Clarksburg, W.V.

Chief Richard Wiederhold, Brevard County Fire and Rescue, Merritt Island, FL.

LAURENCE W. SCHLANGER, M.D.
ER Physician, Good Samaritan Hospital,
West Palm Beach, Florida
Medical Director, InterCity EMS

ABOUT THE AUTHORS

Brent Braunworth, coauthor, is presently employed as a Firefighter–Paramedic for the West Palm Beach Fire Department in Palm Beach County, Florida. He has been a writer for 14 years, having had over 100 articles and short stories published both locally and nationally.

Albert L. Howe, co-author, is presently employed as the Paramedic Program Director at Palm Beach Community College in Lake Worth, Florida. He is a registered nurse with 12 years emergency room experience. He is also licensed in the state of Florida as a paramedic. He has been teaching and coordinating ACLS, BCLS, BTLS, PHTLS and EMT programs for 8 years.

David A. Summers, who set up and photographed the scenes, is a Trauma Resuscitation Nurse for a level 2 trauma center in Palm Beach County. He is also a volunteer Firefighter–Paramedic for Palm Beach County Fire Rescue. He specializes in nature and medical photography and frequently takes rescue scene pictures.

INTRODUCTION

This text is designed to allow various levels of prehospital care providers to experience realistic scenarios. The format is presented in the following manner:

PHOTO
INITIAL SCENE DESCRIPTION
A. DISPATCH INFORMATION
B. SCENE
PRIMARY ASSESSMENT FINDINGS
SECONDARY ASSESSMENT FINDINGS
SCENARIO PROGRESSION AND ANALYSIS
SUGGESTED TREATMENT
A. EMT-A LEVEL TREATMENT
B. EMT-I LEVEL TREATMENT
C. EMT-P LEVEL TREATMENT
ADDITIONAL PROBLEMS SUMMARY

Although this general format is suggested, appropriate *local protocols* must always be taken into consideration and substituted when necessary. The scenarios can involve more than one problem at the presenter's discretion. The scenarios are not meant to be hard and fast in their presentation; each must be presented with flexibility to respond to the candidate's direction of treatment. The presenter should review the summary prior to each scenario presentation so that he or she will be fully aware of the purpose of the scenario.

All scenarios have been written to include three rescuers, although in practice only one candidate is usually tested, the team leader. This does not mean that the whole team cannot be evaluated with this text. Also, if less rescuers are normally used, then adjustments can be made accordingly by the presenter to make allowances for this.

The *photo page* is to be used to help visualize the initial scene. It can be utilized to prepare a simulated scene for the candidates or to help the presenter to describe the scene verbally. Its use is not required, but it is a useful tool to help set the scene for scenario presentation.

The initial scene is comprised of *dispatch information* and scene information. The dispatch information should be read to the candidate before he or she enters the scene or prior to the beginning of testing. This information can utilize local streets and/or areas. This approach may be useful in testing the candidate's knowledge of local areas (zones, maps, or running cards). After the candidate enters the scene or begins the test, the *scene information* should be read to the candidate verbatim.

The *assessment findings* are to be provided as the student conducts each type of survey. If the candidate fails to request a piece of information, the information should be withheld until scenario completion. This will help the presenter to summarize the scenario and critique the performance of the candidate. Even if this information is critical to the patient outcome, it should only be provided if requested. This action can be used as a teaching step in the scenario. Some information found in the primary assessment will be repeated in the secondary assessment in order to be thorough.

Certain abbreviations and pneumonics are used in the scenario format. The presenter must be aware of their meaning before presentation.

- ▼ A = alert
- ▼ V = verbally responsive
- ▼ P = responsive to pain
- ▼ U = unresponsive

- ▼ A = allergies
- ▼ M = medications
- ▼ P = past medical history
- ▼ L = last oral intake
- ▼ E = events leading up to the incident

The *scenario progression and analysis* portion helps the presenter to allow the scenario to flow in a specific direction. It also allows the presenter to incorporate any of the provided additional problems that he or she may see fit to use. This does not mean that the presenter cannot elect to take the scenario in another direction, if so chosen. This section is provided only as a guide.

The *suggested treatment* portion is divided into the Nationally recognized levels of emergency medical prehospital care providers. Some areas may not have all of these levels and the treatment should be modified accordingly. Some scenarios may not be applicable to each level and should be tailored to the level of each candidate. This portion is set up so that some part of the treatment that would be rendered by the EMT-A would also be expected and included in treatment by the EMT-I. The EMT-P section includes all the suggested treatment for paramedics in a step by step list. Although the treatment is given in a step by step format, the presenter should realize that , many times certain types of treatment intervention will be done simultaneously.

In all cases, the presenter must take into consideration local protocols and realize that this portion must be flexible and used only as a guideline. The presenter should change the scenario to meet local needs, with additions or deletions where applicable.

As the candidate performs his or her treatment, the presenter should check against the listed suggested treatment to assure timeliness of intervention. Once the candidate reaches a certain point in the scenario and the patient's condition must change or information must be given, capitalized DIRECTIONS are given to let the presenter have enough time to change the course of the scenario. The authors recommend stating the DIRECTIONS to the candidate once this point is reached. However, the DIRECTIONS in parentheses are for the presenter only; they let him or her know the condition of the patient before the time when the candidate asks. This is how the authors use this area, but it is up to the presenter, after a review of the scenario prior to the presentation, to decide what he wants to say or not.

If there are no DIRECTIONS it means that if the proper treatment is accomplished then the vital signs of the patient should remain the same as the initial findings. If improper treatment is done, it is wholly up to the presenter's discretion whether or not to leave the suggested treatment portion and continue to test the candidate. The authors could not provide a section to cover improper treatment, since there is so much room for error. So, ultimately, it is up to the presenter to determine where to take the candidate (or whether to pass or fail him or her) during the course of the scenario, if the candidate's management varies from what is recommended.

The *additional problems* section is designed to add some flexibility to each scenario and to vary the level of challenge for each scenario use. This section should be utilized to make each scenario applicable on more than one occasion simply by modifying the problems. If the presenter notes that the candidate deals easily with the incorporated problems, he or she can simply increase the difficulty of the scenario by adding problems during the course of the scenario.

The *summary* allows the presenter to explain the scenario in an organized fashion. This section can also be used during the critique of a performance to help compare the suggested treatment to the actions of the candidate. There are also explanations of pathophysiology for the suggested treatment to help summarize the purpose and goals of a particular scenario for the candidate.

Chapter 1

CARDIAC SCENARIOS

CARDIAC SCENARIO 1

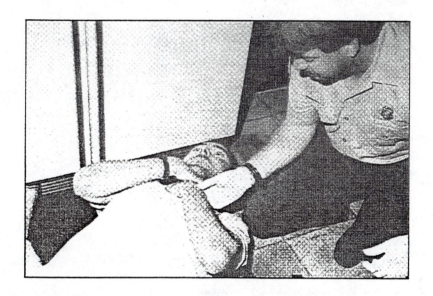

Type: Combination—respiratory, cardiac
Scenario moulage prop list: Live model or mannequin, live model for wife's role,
grease paint or talc for ashen gray skin color, rum or whiskey for alcohol on breath
(kitchen setting)

INITIAL SCENE DESCRIPTION

Dispatch Information

LOCATION: Residential home
NUMBER OF VICTIMS: 1
TYPE OF SITUATION: Man choking
HAZARDS: None
WEATHER CONDITIONS: Warm, clear evening
TIME OF DAY: 1900 hours

Scene

You quickly arrive at the scene; ironically, you were eating dinner right around the corner. As you enter the house, the patient's wife explains that her husband, a 47–year–old male, had been drinking beer and eating dinner when he began to "choke on a piece of chicken." He then "fell out" just before you arrived. The patient is lying prone on the kitchen floor and is arousable by pain at this time.

PRIMARY ASSESSMENT FINDINGS

SCENE SURVEY

▾ residential house
▾ man supine on floor
▾ no apparent hazards

AIRWAY/CERVICAL SPINE

▾ airway obstructed
▾ no signs of trauma
▾ neck veins slightly distended

BREATHING

▾ 0 breaths per minute
▾ exaggerated respiratory effort noted with no ventilation
▾ no chest rise

CIRCULATION/HEMORRHAGE CONTROL

▾ slow, weak carotid pulse at 44
▾ slow, weak radial pulse at 44
▾ capillary refill delayed to 4 seconds
▾ no obvious external blood loss

DISABILITY

▾ (A, V, P, U) responsive only to pain

EXPOSE AND EXAMINE

▾ no obvious deformity or discoloration
▾ skin turgor good
▾ skin color ashen and dusky gray
▾ skin cool and dry to touch
▾ weight estimated at 200 lb

SECONDARY ASSESSMENT FINDINGS

VITAL SIGNS

▾ respirations, 0, effort without effective ventilation
▾ pulse, 44

- ▾ blood pressure, 80/58
- ▾ ECG, a sinus bradycardia

HISTORY

- ▾ as above, except for the following:
    - ▾ A   none
    - ▾ M   none
    - ▾ P   none
    - ▾ L   piece of chicken, beer
    - ▾ E   drinking, eating, and choking

HEAD

- ▾ no visible trauma
- ▾ no deformity on palpation
- ▾ pupils equal and reactive to light

NECK

- ▾ trachea midline
- ▾ neck veins slightly distended
- ▾ no deformity
- ▾ no discoloration

CHEST

- ▾ no visible deformity
- ▾ no chest wall movement
- ▾ no lung sounds
- ▾ no deformity, tenderness, or crepitus on palpation
- ▾ (if checked, heart sounds normal)

ABDOMEN

- ▾ abdomen nondistended
- ▾ soft, nontender to palpation
- ▾ (if checked, bowel sounds present)
- ▾ pelvic rock stable

EXTREMITIES

- ▾ no deformity
- ▾ no discoloration
- ▾ no visible signs of trauma
- ▾ capillary refill delayed to 4 seconds

- slow, weak distal pulses palpated
- skin turgor good
- skin ashen and dusky gray
- skin cool and dry to touch
- no tenderness, crepitus, or swelling
- movement of extremities equal

NEUROLOGICAL

- obtunded, responsive to pain, cannot speak due to obstructed airway
- Glasgow coma scale calculated at 7:
    - eye opening, to pain (2)
    - verbal response is none (1)
    - motor response, withdraws (4)

SENSORY EXAM

- withdraws from painful stimuli and moves all extremities

BACK

- no deformity
- no discoloration
- no trauma noted

Scenario Progression and Analysis: This patient is in respiratory arrest due to a totally obstructed airway. EMT–As and Is will have some success in clearing the airway with abdominal thrusts. This scenario requires repeated application of techniques used to clear the airway and recognition of changes in the patient's airway status. The paramedics will have to perform either a cricothyrotomy or a transtracheal jet insufflation to get a patent airway. EMT–As and Is should be tested on how quickly they diagnose the problem, perform the abdominal thrusts (as per American Heart Association guidelines), control the airway, and eventually perform CPR since this patient will go into cardiac arrest. They must then make the decision to transport or call for an ALS Unit. For the paramedics, even if ACLS guidelines are followed, the patient will continue to deteriorate. This patient will go from a sinus bradycardia to a multitude of different rhythms, finally remaining in asystole.

SUGGESTED TREATMENT

EMT–A Level

- Conduct Scene Survey.
- Conduct Primary Assessment.

▼ Airway management should include proper application of the bag–valve–mask device with 100% O_2 administration.
  ▼ Position patient properly.
  ▼ Open airway with head–tilt, chin–lift.
  ▼ Insert naso/oropharyngeal airway.
  ▼ Ventilate 2 times.

NO RISE IN CHEST NOTED.

▼ Reposition and reventilate.

NO CHEST RISE NOTED.

▼ Perform 5 abdominal thrusts.
  ▼ Examine mouth for obstruction.
  ▼ Perform finger sweep.
  ▼ Reposition and reventilate.

SOME CHEST RISE NOTED.

▼ Complete Primary Assessment.

AT THIS TIME, THE PATIENT IS APENIC WITH A PULSE OF 44 BPM.

▼ Hyperventilate patient.
▼ Insert naso/oropharyngeal airway.
  ▼ Assess lung sounds.
▼ Transport ASAP or call for an ALS Unit.
▼ Conduct Secondary Assessment.

THE PATIENT IS NOW PULSELESS.

▼ Initiate proper CPR.
  ▼ 5 to 1 ratio of compressions to ventilations.
  ▼ 80 to 100 compressions per minute.
  ▼ Proper hand placement and depth of compression.

AT THIS TIME THERE IS NO CHEST RISE WITH VENTILATIONS.

▼ Reposition and reventilate.

STILL NO CHEST RISE.

▼ Perform 5 abdominal thrusts.
  ▼ examine mouth for obstruction.

- ▼ Perform finger sweep.
- ▼ Reposition and reventilate.

SOME CHEST RISE NOTED WITH VENTILATIONS.

- ▼ Reassess airway, breathing, circulation, and level of consciousness.
- ▼ Continue CPR with constant pulse checks with and without compressions.
- ▼ Complete Secondary Assessment.

EMT–I Level

- ▼ Treatment is the same as above, but includes the following:
- ▼ Apply automatic external defibrillator, as per local protocols.
- ▼ Establish a large–bore IV, infusing normal saline or Ringer's lactate, KVO.

EMT–P Level

- ▼ Conduct Scene Survey.
- ▼ Conduct Primary Assessment.
- ▼ Airway management should include proper application of the bag–valve–mask device with 100% O_2 administration.
    - ▼ Position patient properly.
    - ▼ Open airway with head–tilt, chin–lift.
    - ▼ Insert naso/oropharyngeal airway.
    - ▼ Ventilate 2 times.

NO RISE IN CHEST NOTED.

Reposition and reventilate.

NO CHEST RISE NOTED.

Perform 5 abdominal thrusts.
- ▼ Examine mouth for obstruction.
- ▼ Reposition and reventilate.
- ▼ Attempt to visualize and remove the obstruction with forceps.

FOOD IS VISUALIZED. UNABLE TO
REMOVE OBSTRUCTION.

Attempt to ventilate.

NO CHEST RISE.

- ▼ Perform cricothyrotomy or transtracheal jet insufflation as per standing orders.

- ▾ Assess lung sounds.
- ▾ Complete Primary Assessment.

CHEST RISE NOTED NOW. (PATIENT REMAINS APNEIC WITH A PULSE OF 44 BPM.)

- ▾ Hyperventilate patient.
- ▾ Assess ECG, showing a sinus bradycardia.
- ▾ Conduct Secondary Assessment
- ▾ Establish a large bore IV, infusing normal saline or Ringer's lactate, KVO.
- ▾ Administer 0.5 to 1 mg of atropine, IV and repeat every 3 to 5 minutes, as needed, up to 3 mg (or 0.4 mg/kg up to 3 mg).
- ▾ Reassess ECG, airway, breathing, circulation, and level of consciousness.
- ▾ Administer a dopamine drip (or epinephrine drip depending on patient's hypotension) as per local protocols.

AT THIS TIME, THE PATIENT IS PULSELESS. (ECG REVEALS AN IDIOVENTRICULAR RHYTHM OF 30 BPM.)

- ▾ Initiate proper CPR.
    - ▾ 5 to 1 ratio of compressions to ventilations.
    - ▾ 80 to 100 compressions per minute.
    - ▾ proper hand placement and depth of compression.
- ▾ Administer 1 mg of epinephrine, 1:10,000, IV, every 3 to 5 minutes while the patient is pulseless.
- ▾ (New ACLS guidelines suggest that higher doses of epinephrine may be administered in lieu of low doses if these are ineffecive. Local protocols should dictate the amount to be given at the next interval.)
- ▾ Reassess ECG, airway, breathing, circulation, and level of consciousness.
- ▾ Apply pacemaker and reassess ECG and pulse.

CAPTURE IS NEVER OBTAINED.

THE PATIENT REMAINS PULSELESS AND COARSE V–FIB IS NOTED ON THE MONITOR.

- ▾ Check leads, consider precordial thump and reassess, if given.
- ▾ Defibrillate at 200 joules and reassess ECG.
- ▾ Defibrillate at 300 joules and reassess ECG and pulse.

ECG NOW REVEALS ASYSTOLE.

- ▾ Confirm in two leads.
- ▾ Continue CPR with constant pulse checks with and without compressions.

- ▼ Administer 1 mg of epinephrine, 1:10,000, IV, or administer 1 mg of atropine, depending on previous dose given.
- ▼ Reassess ECG, airway, breathing, circulation, and level of consciousness

BREATH SOUNDS ABSENT ON RIGHT SIDE. (HYPER-RESONANCE NOTED ON PERCUSSION.)

- ▼ Reassess lung sounds to confirm catheter or cricothyrotomy tube placement.

BREATH SOUNDS STILL ABSENT ON RIGHT.

- ▼ Continue CPR.
- ▼ Decompress right side of chest, as per local protocols.
- ▼ Reassess ECG, airway, breathing, circulation, and level of consciousness.

BREATH SOUNDS ARE NOW PRESENT, BUT ECG NOW REVEALS A COARSE V–FIB.

- ▼ Check leads and defibrillate at 360 joules and reassess ECG and pulse.

ECG AGAIN REVEALS ASYSTOLE.

- ▼ Confirm in two leads.
- ▼ Continue CPR.
- ▼ Administer 1 mg of epinephrine ,1:10,000, IV.
- ▼ Reassess ECG, airway, breathing, circulation, and level of consciousness.
- ▼ Apply pacemaker and reassess ECG and pulse.

ECG REVEALS PACER SPIKES (WITHOUT CAPTURE AND NO PALPABLE PULSES).

- ▼ Consider sodium bicarbonate.
- ▼ Administer 1 mg atropine up to 3 mg, if not yet given.
- ▼ Continue CPR.
- ▼ Transport ASAP.
- ▼ Notify appropriate receiving facility.
- ▼ Complete Secondary Assessment.

ADDITIONAL PROBLEMS

Depending on the level of the candidate, the following problems can be added to the scenario:
1. During this scenario, the patient's rhythm can change into virtually any rhythm the presenter wishes to test.

2. IV therapy may be unavailable, requiring the candidate to use the cricothyrotomy tube for drug therapy.
3. Any history (such as diabetes) can be given initially, but the proper treatment for the history should be followed during the arrest (that is blood drawn, 50% dextrose given).
4. The candidate could be told that this patient is extremely obese, requiring chest thrusts instead of abdominal thrusts.
5. Any location can be given to test the candidate's street or address competency, using local running cards.
6. Any scene hazard can be incorporated, at the presenter's discretion. (This is in addition to or replacement of those already mentioned.)
7. During the scenario, CPR is ineffective requiring a change in compression depth.
8. The patient could vomit initially, requiring the use of a suction device.
9. Incorrect dispatch information, such as on the chief complaint, can be provided.
10. The candidate could get a pulse back when the pacemaker is finally applied.

SUMMARY

The scenario tests the basic life support skills of all candidates. Although the paramedic level has more problems requiring more advanced management, it should be realized that these have been added to make the scenario interesting. But, the basics are always performed first. If these basic techniques are not performed correctly, then this area should be addressed and remedied. The presenter should not lose sight of the fact that this scenario is designed to test the candidate's basic skills more than anything else. Since the patient's condition does not improve, basic life support is required throughout the entire scenario. Consequently, this cardiac arrest should be a reminder of the old EMS adage: *basic life support before advanced life support.*

Advanced airway procedures, like the cricothyrotomy and transtracheal jet insufflation, are rarely seen in the prehospital setting. In this instance, these procedures were the only option available for airway management. Because these skills are so infrequently utilized, they should be practiced and reviewed on a regular basis.

Although the new American Heart Association guidelines for ACLS has included higher doses of epinephrine after failure with the "standard" 1 mg dose (Class IIb: acceptable, possibly helpful) two recent prospective, randomized studies have failed to show a benefit with the higher doses. By research standards, these are the only two studies to date that have evaluated the higher doses of epinephrine.[1]

[1] I.G. Stiell, P.C. Herbert, and B.N. Weitzman, "High–dose Epinephrine in Adult Cardiac Arrest," N Engl J Med 327 (1992), C.G. Brown, D.R. Martine, and P.E. Pepe, "A Comparison of Standard–dose Epinephrine in Cardiac Arrest Outside the Hospital," N Engl J Med 327 (1992), 1051–55.

CARDIAC SCENARIO 2

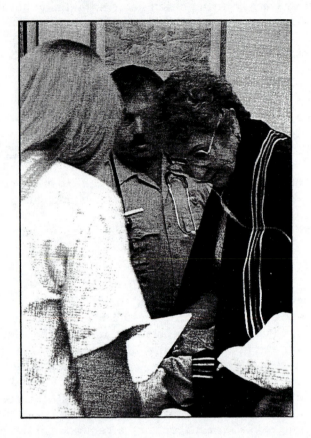

Type: Cardiac, respiratory
Scenario moulage/prop list: Live model or mannequin, live model in nurse's role, chair, grease paint for pale skin color, glycerin water in spray bottle for skin (nursing home setting).

INITIAL SCENE DESCRIPTION

Dispatch Information

LOCATION: Nursing home
NUMBER OF VICTIMS: 1
TYPE OF SITUATION: Shortness of breath
HAZARDS: None
WEATHER CONDITIONS: Warm evening
TIME OF DAY: 1900 hours

Scene

You arrive on scene at a nursing home and are escorted by nurses to the patient's room. There you find a 72–year–old female, sitting up in a chair, in acute respiratory distress. The patient can only nod her head in response to your questions. The nurse explains that she has a COPD and CHF history, but can not tell you her medications at this time. She says she believes she is allergic to sulfa and lidocaine. The patient is breathing 44 times a minute and is on a nasal canula at 2 lpm.

PRIMARY ASSESSMENT FINDINGS

SCENE SURVEY

▾ nursing home room
▾ woman sitting up in chair
▾ no apparent hazards

AIRWAY/CERVICAL SPINE

▾ airway open
▾ no signs of trauma
▾ neck veins distended

BREATHING

▾ 44 breaths per minute, labored and shallow
▾ symmetrical chest rise
▾ rales noted halfway up both lungs

CIRCULATION/HEMORRHAGE CONTROL

▾ irregular carotid pulse at 100
▾ irregular radial pulse at 100
▾ capillary refill delayed to 4 seconds
▾ no obvious external blood loss

DISABILITY

▾ (A, V, P, U) alert

EXPOSE AND EXAMINE

▾ no obvious deformity or discoloration
▾ skin turgor fair
▾ skin color pale

- ▼ skin cool and diaphoretic to touch
- ▼ weight estimated at 160 lb

SECONDARY ASSESSMENT FINDINGS

VITAL SIGNS

- ▼ respirations, 44, labored and shallow
- ▼ pulse, 100 and irregular
- ▼ blood pressure, 88/50
- ▼ ECG, a sinus rhythm with multifocal PVCs

HISTORY

- ▼ as above, except for the following:
  - ▼ A   sulfa, lidocaine
  - ▼ M   unknown
  - ▼ P   COPD, cardiac
  - ▼ L   normal dinner that evening
  - ▼ E   watching TV

HEAD

- ▼ no visible trauma
- ▼ no deformity on palpation
- ▼ pupils equal and reactive to light

NECK

- ▼ trachea midline
- ▼ neck veins distended
- ▼ no deformity
- ▼ no discoloration

CHEST

- ▼ no visible deformity
- ▼ no discoloration
- ▼ symmetrical chest wall movement
- ▼ lung sounds reveal rales midway up both sides
- ▼ no deformity, tenderness, or crepitus on palpation
- ▼ (if checked, heart sounds reveal an S3, S4 gallop)

ABDOMEN

- ▼ abdomen nondistended
- ▼ soft, nontender to palpation

- no masses noted
- (if checked, bowel sounds present)
- pelvic rock stable

EXTREMITIES

- no deformity
- no discoloration
- no visible signs of trauma
- capillary refill delayed to 4 seconds
- distal pulses present
- medical alert bracelet stating an allergy to lidocaine
- skin turgor fair
- skin color pale
- skin cool and diaphoretic to touch
- no tenderness or crepitus
- edema noted to ankles
- movement of extremities equal

NEUROLOGICAL

- conscious, alert
- Glascow coma scale calculated at 15:
    - eye opening, spontaneous (4)
    - verbal response, oriented (5)
    - motor response, obeys (6)

SENSORY EXAM

- no deficit in sensory or motor function

BACK

- no deformity
- no discoloration
- no trauma noted

Scenario Progression and Analysis: This patient is in acute respiratory distress due to congestive heart failure. EMT–As and Is should be evaluated on their rapid diagnosis of the problem, the proper airway control, and the decision to transport and call for ALS assistance. The paramedics should be tested on how quickly they diagnose the problem, properly control the airway, address the hypotension, and initiate the proper treatment to reduce the fluid in her lungs. The paramedics should be aware that furosemide is a sulfonamide and in those patients who are sensitive to sulfa it may cause allergic reactions. However, this incidence of crossover is very small and the benefits of treatment in this case would outweigh the risks. Local protocols should direct the correct care in these kinds of cases. The patient is also allergic to lidocaine, requiring the use of other antidysrhythmic agents. Once the treatment for the airway is complete, the candidate should next raise the blood pressure of the patient to an acceptable level, then address the heart failure, and, finally, treat the PVCs on the monitor. If both the diagnosis and treatment are completed rapidly, the patient's condition will improve. If not, this patient's condition should deteriorate.

SUGGESTED TREATMENT

EMT–A Level

- ▼ Conduct Scene Survey.
- ▼ Conduct Primary Assessment.
- ▼ Recognize this as a true respiratory emergency and transport rapidly or call for an ALS Unit.
- ▼ Airway management should include a change to a mask with a high administration of O_2 as per local protocols.
    - ▼ Observe patient's respiratory drive.
- ▼ Reassess airway, breathing, circulation, and level of consciousness.
- ▼ Notify appropriate receiving facility.
- ▼ Conduct Secondary Assessment.

EMT–I LEVEL

- ▼ Treatment is the same as above, but includes the following:
- ▼ Apply automatic external defibrillator, as per local protocols.
- ▼ Establish a large–bore IV of normal saline or Ringer's lactate, as per local protocols.

EMT–P LEVEL

- ▼ Conduct Scene Survey.
- ▼ Conduct Primary Assessment.
- ▼ Airway management should include a change to a high administration of O_2 with a mask.
- ▼ Assess ECG, showing a sinus rhythm with multifocal PVCs.
- ▼ Establish 1 large–bore IV of normal saline or Ringer's lactate, KVO.
- ▼ Conduct Secondary Assessment.

PATIENT'S BP = 88/50.

- ▼ Administer dopamine, as per local protocols.
- ▼ Reassess ECG, airway, breathing, circulation, and level of consciousness.

PATIENT'S BP = 118/70.

- ▼ Administer furosemide, as per local protocols.
- ▼ Reassess airway, breathing, circulation, and level of consciousness.
- ▼ Administer morphine, as per local protocols.
- ▼ Reassess airway, breathing, circulation, and level of consciousness.
- ▼ Administer nitroglycerin, as per local protocols.
- ▼ Reassess airway, breathing, circulation, and level of consciousness.

PATIENT'S BREATHING SLOWS TO 28 BREATHS PER MINUTE (WHILE LUNG SOUNDS ARE NOW CLEAR ON THE LEFT). ECG IS STILL SHOWING MULTIFOCAL PVC'S.

- ▼ Administer 20 mg/min. (may give up to 30 mg/min.) bolus of procainamide, as per local protocols up to a total of 17 mg/kg.
- ▼ Reassess ECG, airway, breathing, circulation, and level of consciousness.

ECG = A NORMAL SINUS RHYTHM WITHOUT PVC'S.

- ▼ Administer a procainamide drip at a 1:4 ratio, infusing at 1 to 4 mg/min.
- ▼ Transport ASAP.
- ▼ Notify appropriate receiving facility.

ADDITIONAL PROBLEMS

Depending on the level of the candidate, the following problems can be added to the scenario:

1. The patient may experience cardiac dysrhythmias due to the administration of the dopamine.
2. The patient's hypotension may continue after the initial administration of the dopamine, requiring a higher dosage.
3. The presenter may wish to cause the patient to have an allergic reaction that the candidate must treat, following the administration of the furosemide.
4. The patient may have increased hypotension or widening of the QRS by 50% from procainamide, requiring another antidysrhythmic.
5. Even though the correct medications are given, the patient may still go into cardiac arrest.
6. The patient's lungs might not clear up immediately, requiring that another bolus of furosemide, or morphine, be given.
7. Following the administration of morphine, the patient can experience profound hypotension and/or respiratory depression, requiring intubation and naloxone to reverse the effect.

8. The patient may experience a decrease in level of consciousness and respirations after the administration of high–flow O_2 due to suppression of the patient's respiratory drive.

10. Any scene hazard can be incorporated, at the presenter's discretion. (This is in addition to or replacement of those already mentioned.)

11. If a pulse oximeter reading is asked for by the candidate, an appropriate reading should be given.

SUMMARY

This patient has a past history of COPD and congestive heart failure. Chronic obstructive pulmonary disease causes an increase in pressure in the pulmonary circulation. This constant increased resistance that the right heart must pump against can lead to right ventricular enlargement and eventual pump failure. Right heart failure may cause left ventricular failure. These patients have a very tenuous volume status already, and any additional fluid or decrease in the pump's effectiveness will place them in cardiogenic shock with pulmonary edema. The treatment should be directed toward the reduction of the preload (the amount of blood returning to the right heart) and the reduction of afterload (the resistance that the left heart must pump against). Morphine mildly reduces both preload and afterload, as well as being effective in reducing any pain and anxiety that the patient may be experiencing. Both pain and anxiety can result in the release of catacholamines, which will increase the heart rate and the afterload. These will increase the oxygen demand of the myocardium and could cause further loss of the pump's effectiveness. Nitroglycerin is much more effective than morphine in reducing preload and afterload, as well as for dilating the coronary arteries and increasing oxygen availability for the myocardium.

The patient history also includes an allergy to sulfonamides. This is a common allergy, so the prehospital care provider needs to be aware that this group of drugs includes not only antibiotics, but also furosemide. Patients who have developed sensitivity to the antibiotics may be sensitive to the diuretic Cross–sensitivity is rare, but some physicians feel that furosemide should not be administered to patients with a sulfonamide allergy. In this case, local protocols should dictate candidates' actions.

The paramedic should first consider the patient's blood pressure when administering any of the above drugs, since all can cause hypotension. In this case the blood pressure was addressed before their administration. The initial dose of dopamine will increase the cardiac output by increasing the force of contraction, as well as the heart rate. It will also cause vasoconstriction at higher doses, which can also increase blood pressure . Once the blood pressure is above 90 mm Hg , morphine and nitroglycerin can be administered.

The patient also has a history of lidocaine sensitivity. The incidence of true lidocaine sensitivity is, again, rare, but many physicians feel that if the patient states a history of this allergy, lidocaine should not be administered. The author chose to administer a second–line antidysrhythmic drug, procainamide. Thi drug cannot be administered until after the hypotension has been addressed since it can cause hypotension as well.

The suggested treatment for EMT–As and Is calls for the administration of a high concentration of oxygen. These providers are frequently taught that this should not be done in the patient with a history of COPD because of concern for suppressing the hypoxic drive, resulting in CO_2 retention and severe acidosis. This is a possibility, but only about 4% of all COPD patients have true hypoxic drive. This may be a concern in some hospital emergency rooms, where a patient may not be seen for some length of time, but the prehospital care provider should normally not be so concerned about this. Since prehospital providers are constantly reassessing their patients, any change in level of consciousness would be noted and the oxygen concentration could be reduced. If the respiratory drive was suppressed, then the provider could always support respirations until advance airway procedures could be instituted. In most locales, the transport time is shorter than the time required to suppress the hypoxic drive found in the COPD patient.

CARDIAC SCENARIO 3

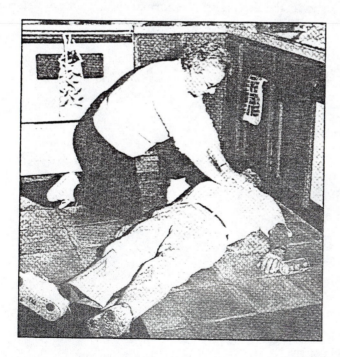

Type Cardiac.
Scenario moulage/prop list: Live model or mannequin, live model for wife's role, grease paint for pale skin color, glycerin water for skin, labeled pill bottles, unfinished breakfast on table (kitchen setting).

INITIAL SCENE DESCRIPTION

Dispatch Information

LOCATION: Suburban home
NUMBER OF VICTIMS: 1
TYPE OF SITUATION: Man down
HAZARDS: None
WEATHER CONDITIONS: Cool fall morning
TIME OF DAY: 0730 hours

Scene

Upon arrival to a suburban residence you find a 70–year–old male patient supine in the kitchen area. His wife is providing what appears to be effective CPR at this time. Your partners begin BLS and question the patient's wife as you prepare the defibrillator. The wife is upset but begins to explain that her husband has an extensive cardiac and hypertensive history and "just got out of the hospital last week." He was hospitalized for an acute myocardial infarction. With the quick–look mode, the ECG reveals a normal sinus rhythm. You reassess a carotid pulse without CPR in progress and find none present. His color is mottled and his skin is cool to the touch. You advise your partner to continue CPR as you begin treatment.

PRIMARY ASSESSMENT FINDINGS

SCENE SURVEY

- ▼ suburban home kitchen area
- ▼ unfinished breakfast on the table
- ▼ no apparent hazards

AIRWAY/CERVICAL SPINE

- ▼ airway closed with tongue obstruction
- ▼ no signs of trauma
- ▼ neck veins distended

BREATHING

- ▼ no spontaneous breathing noted
- ▼ no chest rise

CIRCULATION/HEMORRHAGE CONTROL

- ▼ no carotid pulse
- ▼ no radial pulse

- ▼ capillary refill delayed and immeasurable
- ▼ no obvious external blood loss

DISABILITY

- ▼ **(A, V, P, U) UNRESPONSIVE**

EXPOSE AND EXAMINE

- ▼ no obvious deformity or discoloration
- ▼ skin color mottled
- ▼ skin turgor fair
- ▼ skin cool and diaphoretic to touch
- ▼ estimated weight at 200 lb

SECONDARY ASSESSMENT FINDINGS

VITAL SIGNS

- ▼ respirations, 0
- ▼ pulse, 0
- ▼ blood pressure, 0/0
- ▼ ECG, a sinus rhythm with a rate of 100

HISTORY

- ▼ as above, except for the following:
  - ▼ A   none
  - ▼ M   metoprolol, aspirin, alprazolam, nitro–dur
  - ▼ P   angina, one acute myocardial infarction 2 weeks prior, hypertension
  - ▼ L   partial breakfast
  - ▼ E   eating breakfast, complained of chest pain, suddenly lost consciousness and the wife started CPR immediately

HEAD

- ▼ no visible trauma
- ▼ no deformity on palpation
- ▼ pupils equal, dilated and fixed

NECK

- ▼ trachea midline
- ▼ neck veins distended
- ▼ no deformity
- ▼ no discoloration

CHEST

- no visible deformity
- no discoloration
- symmetrical chest wall movement with respiratory support
- lung sounds clear and equal, bilaterally with supported ventilations
- no deformity, tenderness ,or crepitus on palpation (if checked, heart sounds muffled and distant)

ABDOMEN

- abdomen nondistended
- soft, nontender to palpation
- no masses noted
- (if checked, bowel sounds absent)
- pelvic rock stable

EXTREMITIES

- no deformity
- no discoloration
- no visual signs of trauma
- capillary refill delayed and immeasurable
- no distal pulses present
- skin turgor fair
- skin color mottled
- skin cool and diaphoretic to touch
- no tenderness, crepitus, or swelling
- no movement of extremities

NEUROLOGICAL

- unconscious, unresponsive
- Glascow coma scale calculated at 3:
    - eye opening, none (1)
    - verbal response, none (1)
    - motor response, none (1)

SENSORY EXAM

- unable to determine sensory or motor function

BACK

- no deformity
- no discoloration
- no trauma noted

Scenario Progression and Analysis: CPR was initiated almost immediately and, of course, on arrival should continue. The rhythm should be recognized as PEA (Pulseless with electrical activity) and treated as per local protocols and AHA algorithms. EMT–As should be tested on how quickly they diagnose cardiac arrest, perform proper CPR, and transport or call for an ALS Unit. EMT-Is should be tested the same as the paramedics. This should include rapid assessment and transportation. For the paramedics, if proper ACLS guidelines are followed, then this patient will have the rhythm remain the same, but pulses will return with a fluid challenge and antishock trouser application. If the rhythm is not treated correctly, the patient will develop ventricular fibrillation midway through the treatment, converting then to an asystolic rhythm, and will consequently be unresponsive to treatment.

SUGGESTED TREATMENT

EMT–A Level

- ▼ Conduct Scene Survey.
- ▼ Conduct Primary Assessment.
- ▼ Recognize the cardiac nature of this patient and transport rapidly or call for ALS personnel.
- ▼ Airway management should include proper application of the bag–valve–mask device with 100% O_2 administration.
  - ▼ Position patient properly.
  - ▼ Open airway with head–tilt, chin–lift.
  - ▼ Insert naso/oropharyngeal airway.
- ▼ Initiate proper CPR.
  - ▼ 5 to 1 ratio of compressions to ventilations.
  - ▼ 80 to 100 compressions per minute.
  - ▼ Proper hand placement and depth of compression.
- ▼ Reassess airway, breathing, circulation, and level of consciousness.
- ▼ Notify appropriate receiving facility.
- ▼ Conduct Secondary Assessment.

EMT–I Level

- ▼ Treatment is the same as above but includes the following:
- ▼ Apply external automatic defibrillator ASAP, or as per local protocols.
- ▼ Airway management should include insertion of an esophageal airway.
  - ▼ Place in sniffing position.
  - ▼ Assess lung sounds.
- ▼ Apply the pneumatic antishock garment, as per local protocols.
- ▼ Reassess ECG, airway, breathing, circulation, and level of consciousness.

- ▼ Establish one large–bore IV, infusing Ringer's lactate, open, as per local protocols.
- ▼ Reassess airway, breathing, circulation, and level of consciousness.

EMT–P Level

- ▼ Conduct Scene Survey.
- ▼ Conduct Primary Assessment, which includes a rapid ECG assessment, showing a normal sinus rhythm.
- ▼ Airway management should include proper application of the bag–valve–mask device with 100% O_2 administration.
  - ▼ Position patient properly.
  - ▼ Open airway with head–tilt, chin–lift.
  - ▼ Insert naso/oropharyngeal airway.
- ▼ Initiate proper CPR.
  - ▼ 5 to 1 ratio of compressions to ventilations.
  - ▼ 80 to 100 compressions per minute.
  - ▼ Proper hand placement and depth of compression.
- ▼ Complete oral intubation with appropriate–sized tube.
  - ▼ Hyperventilate before and after.
  - ▼ No longer than 30 seconds.
  - ▼ Assess lung sounds.
- ▼ Reassess ECG, airway, breathing, circulation, and level of consciousness.
- ▼ Establish a large–bore IV, infusing normal saline or Ringer's lactate, KVO.
- ▼ Administer 1 mg of epinephrine, 1:10,000, IV, every 3 to 5 minutes while the patient is pulseless.
- ▼ (New ACLS guidelines suggest that higher doses of epinephrine may be administered in lieu of low doses if these are ineffective. Local protocols should dictate the amount to be given at the next interval.)
- ▼ Reassess ECG, airway, breathing, circulation, and level of consciousness.
- ▼ Conduct Secondary Assessment and consider the causes for being pulseless with electrical activity:
  - ▼ Hypovolemia
  - ▼ Hypoxemia
  - ▼ Cardiac tamponade
  - ▼ Tension pneumothorax
  - ▼ Acidosis
  - ▼ Massive pulmonary embolism
  - ▼ Hypothermia
  - ▼ Hyperkalemia
  - ▼ Drug overdoses
  - ▼ Massive AMI
- ▼ Assure lung sounds are clear and equal with ventilation.

- ▼ Hyperventilate patient and reassess.
- ▼ Initiate a fluid bolus with either Ringer's lactate or normal saline of 200 cc, as per local protocols.
  - ▼ Assess lung sounds.
- ▼ Reassess ECG, airway, breathing, circulation, and level of consciousness.

**AT THE NEXT PULSE CHECK WITHOUT CPR, A
WEAK, CORRESPONDING CAROTID PULSE (OF 100)
SHOULD BE PALPATED. ECG STILL REVEALS
A NORMAL SINUS RHYTHM.**

- ▼ Repeat another bolus to assure this to be hypovolemia.
- ▼ Reassess ECG, airway, breathing, circulation, and level of consciousness.

**PATIENT'S CAROTID PULSE BECOMES STRONGER.
PATIENT'S BP STILL CANNOT BE AUSCULTATED.**

- ▼ Apply the pneumatic antishock garment, as per local protocols.
- ▼ Reassess ECG, airway, breathing, circulation, and level of consciousness.

PATIENT'S BP = 60/40.

- ▼ Transport ASAP.
- ▼ Establish second large–bore IV, infusing either Ringer's lactate or normal saline, open.
- ▼ Reassess ECG airway, breathing, circulation, and level of consciousness.
- ▼ Notify appropriate receiving facility.

ADDITIONAL PROBLEMS

Depending on the level of the candidate, the following problems can be added to the scenario:

1. During the scenario, CPR is ineffective, requiring a change in compression depth.
2. Before the defibrillator arrives, have the candidate perform one–person CPR
3. Any history (such as diabetes) can be given initially, but the proper treatment for the history should be followed during the arrest (that is, blood drawn, 50% dextrose given).
4. During airway management, the endotracheal tube placement can take too long or be improperly placed in the right bronchus. It can also never be placed in the trachea, requiring the candidate to insert an esophageal airway.

5. The patient can also remain pulseless having developed a tension pneumothorax requiring chest decompression

6. The Candidate can have difficulty in IV insertion, so the pneumatic anti-shock garment should be used, initially, to rule out hypovolemia.

7. The patient does not respond to the fluid infusions, requiring the candidate to continue on with ACLS protocols, and the like.

8. Any location can be given to test the candidate's street or address competency, using local running cards.

9. Any scene hazard can be incorporated at the presenter's discretion. (This is in addition to or replacement of those already mentioned.)

SUMMARY

This patient is suffering from a ventricular aneurysm, causing a ventricular rupture and profound hypovolemia, presenting all the signs and symptoms of cardiac tamponade. This is most commonly seen in women and hypertensives in their seventh decade. Approximately 10 days to 2 weeks following an acute myocardial infarction, a weakening of the ventricular wall (due to necrosis) at the site of the infarction can occur. This can most likely be seen by prehospital personnel after someone has been released from hospital admissions 2 or 3 weeks before. There may be no other symptom, other than a sudden cardiac arrest. Once PEA is noted on the monitor and guidelines are followed, some of the causes of the PEA should be ruled out. Lung sounds should be checked to rule out a tension pneumothorax, and the patient should be hyperventilated to assure that acidosis or hypoxemia is not the cause of the problem, thus hindering the resuscitation process. A fluid bolus should also be given at this time in order to address the possibility of hypovolemia. Pneumatic antishock trousers can also help to either rule out the cause or aid in the treatment of hypovolemia although its use is controversial. A secondary survey can assist in identifying the cause.

A physical assessment should be performed to evaluate the presence or absence of pericardial tamponade and pulmonary embolus. The appearance of distended neck veins or the auscultation of muffled heart sounds may be the only signs to indicate these two causes of PEA.

CARDIAC SCENARIO 4

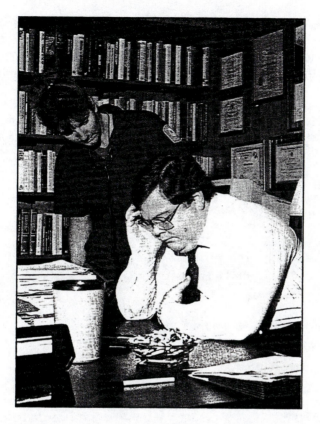

Type: Cardiac
Scenario moulage/prop list: Live obese model or mannequin,
grease paint for mottled skin color, glycerin water for skin, ashtray
full of cigarettes, large coffee cup (office setting).

INITIAL SCENE DESCRIPTION

Dispatch Information

LOCATION: Law office
NUMBER OF VICTIMS: 1
TYPE OF SITUATION: General weakness and dizziness
HAZARDS: None
WEATHER CONDITIONS: Clear
TIME OF DAY: 0930 hours

Scene

You are directed, by a security officer, to a law office on the seventh floor of a large office building downtown. When you arrive you find a 45–year–old male, sitting up leaning on his desk, complaining of a sudden onset of weakness and dizziness. As you question him, he states that he has no medical history other than being "a workaholic, a 3 pack–a–day smoker, and a heavy drinker of cof-fee." This patient is grossly obese at 5 feet 6 inches tall with a weight of 275 pounds. He denies any drug use. Upon scene survey, you see an ashtray filled with cigarette butts and ashes. A large, half–filled cup of coffee sits on his desk.

PRIMARY ASSESSMENT FINDINGS

SCENE SURVEY

- ▼ window office in large office building
- ▼ man sitting up in chair
- ▼ ashtray full of butts and ashes
- ▼ no apparent hazards

AIRWAY/CERVICAL SPINE

- ▼ airway open
- ▼ no signs of trauma
- ▼ neck veins flat

BREATHING

- ▼ 18 breaths per minute, nonlabored
- ▼ symmetrical chest rise
- ▼ lungs clear bilaterally

CIRCULATION/HEMORRHAGE CONTROL

- ▼ carotid pulse too rapid to count
- ▼ radial pulse too rapid to count
- ▼ capillary refill at 3 seconds
- ▼ no obvious external blood loss

DISABILITY

- ▼ (A, V, P, U) alert

EXPOSE AND EXAMINE

- ▼ no obvious deformity or discoloration
- ▼ skin turgor good

- ▼ skin color mottled
- ▼ skin cool and diaphoretic to touch
- ▼ weight estimated at 275 lb

SECONDARY ASSESSMENT FINDINGS

VITAL SIGNS

- ▼ respirations, 18
- ▼ pulse, too rapid to count
- ▼ blood pressure, 160/100
- ▼ ECG, a monomorphic ventricular tachycardia with a rate of 150

HISTORY

- ▼ as above, except for the following:
    - ▼ A   none
    - ▼ M   none
    - ▼ P   heavy smoker, obese
    - ▼ L   coffee and doughnuts
    - ▼ E   working, nonphysical

HEAD

- ▼ no visible trauma
- ▼ no deformity on palpation
- ▼ pupils equal and reactive to light

NECK

- ▼ trachea midline
- ▼ neck veins flat
- ▼ no deformity
- ▼ no discoloration

CHEST

- ▼ no visible deformity
- ▼ no discoloration
- ▼ symmetrical chest wall movement
- ▼ lung sounds clear and equal, bilaterally
- ▼ no deformity, tenderness, or crepitus on palpation
- ▼ (if checked, heart sounds normal)

ABDOMEN

- ▼ abdomen nontender
- ▼ soft, nontender to palpation

▼ if checked, bowel sounds absent)
▼ no masses noted
▼ pelvic rock stable

EXTREMITIES

▼ no deformity
▼ no discoloration
▼ no visible signs of trauma
▼ capillary refill at 3 seconds
▼ distal pulses present
▼ skin turgor good
▼ skin mottled
▼ skin cool and diaphoretic to touch
▼ no tenderness, crepitus ,or swelling
▼ movement of extremities equal

NEUROLOGICAL

▼ conscious, alert
▼ Glascow coma scale calculated at 15:
  ▼ eye opening, spontaneous (4)
  ▼ verbal response, oriented (5)
  ▼ motor response, obeys (6)

SENSORY EXAM

▼ no deficit sensory or motor function

BACK

▼ no deformity
▼ no discoloration
▼ no trauma noted

Scenario Progression and Analysis: This will initially be a patient in a stable ventricular tachycardia. EMT–As and Is should be tested on how quickly they diagnose the problem, initiate the proper treatment, transport, and/or call for help. For the paramedics, once they give lidocaine, the patient will become unstable, with a significant decrease in his level of consciousness and blood pressure. After the first cardioversion, the patient will go into cardiac arrest, remaining in this same rhythm. If ACLS guidelines are followed, this patient will improve and come back into a sinus rhythm. If not, this patient should go into an unresponsive ventricular fibrillation for the scenario's duration.

SUGGESTED TREATMENT

EMT–A Level

▼ Conduct Scene Survey.

▼ Conduct Primary Assessment.

▼ Recognize the cardiac nature of this patient and transport rapidly or call for an ALS Unit.

▼ Airway management should include high–flow O_2 administration with a mask.

▼ Reassess airway, breathing, circulation and level of consciousness.

▼ Conduct Secondary Assessment

AT THIS TIME, THE PATIENT BECOMES EXTREMELY SLUGGISH TO RESPOND (WITH A CAROTID PULSE OF 150 AND RESPIRATIONS AT 32/MINUTE).

▼ Reassess airway, breathing, circulation and level of consciousness.

▼ Airway management should include proper application of the bag–valve–mask device with 100% O_2 administration.
  ▼ Position patient properly.
  ▼ Open airway with head–tilt, chin–lift.
  ▼ Insert naso/oropharyngeal airway.

▼ Notify appropriate receiving facility.

EMT–I Level

▼ Treatment is the same as above, but includes the following:

▼ Apply the automatic external defibrillator, as per local protocols once patient becomes sluggish..

THE AED DEFIBRILLATES REPEATEDLY AND THEN STOPS.

▼ Reassess airway, breathing, circulation, and level of consciousness.

THE PATIENT APPEARS CONSCIOUS AND BREATHING IS WNL.

▼ Continue O_2 therapy and establish a large bore IV, infusing normal saline or Ringer's lactate, KVO.

▼ Place patient in the recovery position.

▼ Transport ASAP.

▼ Conduct Secondary Assessment.

EMT–P Level:

- ▼ Conduct Scene Survey.
- ▼ Conduct Primary Assessment, which includes assessment of ECG, showing ventricular tachycardia.
- ▼ Airway management should include– O_2 administration with a mask.
- ▼ Conduct Secondary Assessment.
- ▼ Establish a large–bore IV infusing normal saline or Ringer's lactate KVO.
- ▼ Recheck allergies to lidocaine and administer 1 to 1.5 mg/kg of lidocaine, IV.
- ▼ Reassess ECG, airway, breathing, circulation, and level of consciousness.

AT THIS TIME, THE PATIENT BECOMES EXTREMELY SLUGGISH WHILE VENTRICULAR TACHYCARDIA REMAINS ON THE MONITOR (WITH A CAROTID PULSE AT 150 AND RESPIRATIONS OF 32/MINUTE).

- ▼ Consider diazepam, 5.0 mg, IV, or as per local protocols.
- ▼ Airway management should include proper application of the bag–valve–mask device with 100% O_2 administration.
  - ▼ Position patient properly.
  - ▼ Open airway with head–tilt, chin–lift.
  - ▼ Insert naso/oropharyngeal airway.
- ▼ Unsynchronized cardioversion at 100 joules should be performed ASAP.
- ▼ Reassess ECG, airway, breathing, circulation, and level of consciousness.

AT THIS TIME THE PATIENT IS APNEIC AND PULSE-LESS, WHILE VENTRICULAR TACHYCARDIA REMAINS ON THE MONITOR.

- ▼ Defibrillate at 200 joules and reassess ECG.
- ▼ Defibrillate at 300 joules and reassess ECG.
- ▼ Defibrillate at 360 joules and reassess ECG and pulse.
- ▼ Initiate proper CPR.
  - ▼ 5 to 1 ratio of compressions to ventilations.
  - ▼ 80 to 100 compressions per minute.
  - ▼ Proper hand placement and depth of compression.
- ▼ Complete oral intubation with appropriate–sized tube.
  - ▼ No longer than 30 seconds.
  - ▼ Assess lung sounds.
- ▼ Administer 1 mg of epinephrine, 1:10,000, IV every 5 minutes while patient is pulseless.
- ▼ (New ACLS guidelines suggest that higher doses of epinephrine may be

administered in lieu of low doses if these are ineffective. Local protocols should dictate the amount to be given at the next interval.)

▼ Confirmation of the rhythm and pulse checks should be constantly assessed with and without compressions.

▼ Defibrillate at 360 joules and reassess ECG and pulse.

AT THIS TIME THE PATIENT'S RHYTHM IS A SINUS TACHYCARDIA WITH A CORRESPONDING PULSE.

▼ Reassess airway, breathing, circulation and level of consciousness.

AT THIS TIME THE PATIENT APPEARS CONSCIOUS, ATTEMPTING TO PULL OUT THE ET TUBE (WHILE RESPIRATIONS APPEAR WNL).

▼ Apply restraints.

▼ Administer a lidocaine drip infusing 1 g at 2 to 4 mg/min.

▼ (The new ACLS standards do not recommend prophylactic lidocaine boluses with the return of a pulse unless PVCs are present. Local protocols should be followed.)

▼ Reassess ECG, airway, breathing, circulation, and level of consciousness. Continue O_2 therapy.

THE PATIENT'S BP = 80 BY PALPATION.

▼ Place patient in Trendelenburg and reassess.

THE PATIENT'S BP = 96/52.

▼ Transport ASAP and conduct Secondary Assessment.

ADDITIONAL PROBLEMS

Depending on the level of the candidate, the following problems can be added to the scenario:

1. During the scenario, just prior to the patient's rhythm change, have the patient vomit.

2. Any history (such as diabetes) can be given initially, but the proper treatment for the history should be followed during the arrest (that is blood drawn, 50% dextrose given).

3. During airway management, the endotracheal tube placement can take too long or be improperly placed in the right bronchus. It can also never be placed in the trachea, requiring the candidate to insert an esophageal airway.

4. The candidate can be taken further down each algorithm before the instructor elects to bring the patient out of ventricular tachycardia.
5. Candidate can have difficulty in IV insertion, requiring that medications be given down the ET tube.
6. Incorrect dispatch information, such as on the chief complaint, can be provided.
7. Any location can be given to test the candidate's street or address competency, using local running cards.
8. Any scene hazard can be incorporated at the presenter's discretion. (This is in addition to or replacement of those already mentioned.)
9. During the scenario, CPR is ineffective, requiring a change in compression depth.
10. This patient could remain hypotensive, requiring the use of dopamine.

SUMMARY

This patient, despite the fact that he had no history of heart disease, did have several modifiable risk factors. Obesity, smoking, and high stress all contribute to heart disease. The incidence of lethal dysrhythmias in patients with no documented preexisting heart disease is noted. The onset of lethal dysrhythmias may be the first sign of a patient's heart disease. Initially, in a stable ventricular tachycardia, drug therapy is attempted before electrical therapy. Lidocaine is indicated to depress phase 4 depolarization of the myocardial cell, reducing reentry and, one hopes, terminating the lethal dysrhythmia. If the patient becomes unstable (chest pain, dyspnea, hypotension, congestive heart failure, ischemia, or infarction), then cardioversion is indicated. If the patient is hypotensive, has pulmonary edema, or loses consciousness, then the cardioversion should be unsynchronized. The rationale behind this being unsynchronized is that the patient is so unstable, normal synchronization might take too long to sense and discharge. This delay could further complicate the termination of this dysrhythmia, since the decreased perfusion causes hypoxia and acidosis.

(Once this patient is pulseless, new ACLS guidelines recommend stacked defibrilations with no pulse checks in between for the same reasons as above.)[2]

[2] "Guidelines for Cardiopulmonary Resuscitation and Emergency Care," JAMA, 268 (1992), No. 16, 2217.

CARDIAC SCENARIO 5

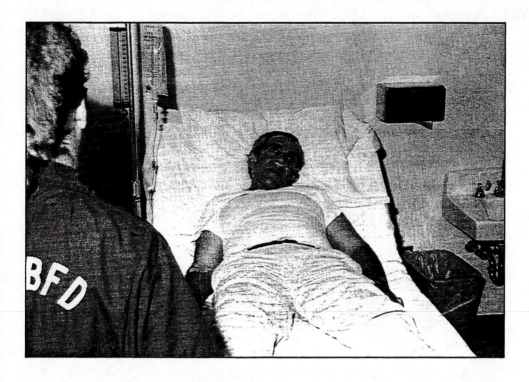

Type: Cardiac

Scenario moulage/prop list: Live model or mannequin, live model for MD's role, grease paint for jaundice skin color, glycerin water for skin, IV with tubing, nasal canula, rum or whiskey for etoh breath (clinic setting).

INITIAL SCENE DESCRIPTION

Dispatch Information

LOCATION: Clinic

NUMBER OF VICTIMS: 1

TYPE OF SITUATION: Chest pain

HAZARDS: None

WEATHER CONDITIONS: Clear

TIME OF DAY: 1630 hours

Scene

It is about 4:30 in the afternoon when you are called to the local clinic for "chest pain." When you arrive, you are directed to a back room where you find a

59–year–old male, sitting up on a bed, complaining of a substernal "pressure" with radiation down his left arm for about 25 minutes. He explains that he's "had this before, but never went to a doctor and never had this so bad." He appears anxious and his skin is cool and diaphoretic to the touch. He states he has no SOB and no medical history other than "liver disease" due to his "drinking."

The physician at the clinic did not have access to an ECG machine, so he "held off on any nitro." They did, however, place him on oxygen at 2 lpm and start an IV of 5% dextrose.

PRIMARY ASSESSMENT FINDINGS

SCENE SURVEY

- ▼ man in bed in back exam room of clinic
- ▼ alcoholic beverage noted on breath
- ▼ no apparent hazards

AIRWAY/CERVICAL SPINE

- ▼ airway open
- ▼ no signs of trauma
- ▼ neck veins slightly distended

BREATHING

- ▼ 28 breaths per minute, slightly labored
- ▼ symmetrical chest rise
- ▼ neck veins distended
- ▼ lungs clear bilaterally

CIRCULATION/HEMORRHAGE CONTROL

- ▼ irregular carotid pulse at 84
- ▼ irregular radial pulse at 84
- ▼ capillary refill at 2 seconds
- ▼ no obvious external blood loss

DISABILITY

- ▼ (A, V, P, U) alert

EXPOSE AND EXAMINE

- ▼ no obvious deformity or discoloration
- ▼ skin turgor fair
- ▼ skin color slightly jaundiced
- ▼ skin cool and diaphoretic to touch
- ▼ weight estimated at 135 lb

SECONDARY ASSESSMENT FINDINGS

VITAL SIGNS

- ▼ respirations, 28
- ▼ pulse, 84 and irregular
- ▼ blood pressure, 178/90
- ▼ ECG, a normal sinus rhythm with multifocal PVCs

HISTORY

- ▼ as above, except for the following:
    - ▼ A none
    - ▼ M none
    - ▼ P alcoholism, liver disease
    - ▼ L none today
    - ▼ E walking

HEAD

- ▼ no visible trauma
- ▼ no deformity on palpation
- ▼ pupils equal and reactive

NECK

- ▼ trachea midline
- ▼ neck veins slightly distended
- ▼ no deformity
- ▼ no discoloration

CHEST

- ▼ no visible deformity
- ▼ symmetrical chest wall movement
- ▼ lung sounds clear and equal
- ▼ no deformity, tenderness, or crepitus on palpation
- ▼ (if checked, heart sounds normal)

ABDOMEN

- ▼ abdomen distended
- ▼ soft, nontender to palpation
- ▼ no masses noted
- ▼ (if checked, bowel sounds present)
- ▼ pelvic rock stable

EXTREMITIES

- ▼ no deformity
- ▼ no discoloration
- ▼ no visible signs of trauma
- ▼ capillary refill at 2 seconds
- ▼ irregular distal pulses present
- ▼ skin turgor fair
- ▼ skin normal color
- ▼ skin cool and diaphoretic to touch
- ▼ no tenderness or crepitus
- ▼ 3+ pedal edema noted bilaterally
- ▼ movement of extremities equal

NEUROLOGICAL

- ▼ conscious, alert
- ▼ Glascow coma scale calculated at 15:
    - ▼ eye opening, spontaneous (4)
    - ▼ verbal response, oriented (5)
    - ▼ motor response, obeys (6)

SENSORY EXAM

- ▼ no deficit in sensory or motor function

BACK

- ▼ no deformity
- ▼ no discoloration
- ▼ no trauma noted

Scenario Progression and Analysis: The patient's problem continues to increase, finally resulting in cardiac arrest. EMT As and Is should be tested on how quickly they diagnose that this is a cardiac emergency, initiate proper treatment, including airway control and eventually CPR, and transport or call for an ALS Unit. For the paramedics, once the initial treatment is done O_2, ECG, IV, and so on), lidocaine should be given IV to clear up the patient's ectopy and nitroglycerin or morphine sulfate given for the chest pain. After this, the patient should continue to have some PVCs and then go into an unstable ventricular tachycardia (with a loss of consciousness) due to the R on T phenomenon. From this rhythm, the patient will almost immediately go into a ventricular fibrillation. If ACLS guidelines are followed, then the patient will improve, converting to a sinus rhythm later. If not, the patient should remain in arrest.

SUGGESTED TREATMENT

EMT–A Level

▼ Conduct Scene Survey.

▼ Conduct Primary Assessment.

▼ Recognize the cardiac nature of this patient and transport rapidly or call for an ALS Unit.

▼ Airway management should include a change to a mask with high– flow O_2 administration.

▼ Reassess airway, breathing, circulation and level of consciousness.

▼ Conduct Secondary Assessment.

AT THIS TIME, THE PATIENT IS APNEIC AND PULSELESS.

▼ Airway management should include proper application of the bag–valve–mask device with 100% O_2 administration.
  - ▼ Position patient properly.
  - ▼ Open airway with head–tilt, chin–lift.
  - ▼ Insert naso/oropharyngeal airway.

▼ Initiate proper CPR.
  - ▼ 5 to 1 ratio of compressions to ventilations.
  - ▼ 80 to 100 compressions per minute.
  - ▼ Proper hand placement and depth of compression.

▼ Reassess airway, breathing, circulation, and level of consciousness.

▼ Notify appropriate receiving facility.

EMT–I LEVEL

▼ Treatment is the same as above, but includes the following:

▼ Apply the automatic external defibrillator, as per local protocols.

▼ Airway management should include insertion of an esophageal airway.
  - ▼ Place in sniffing position.
  - ▼ Assess lung sounds.

▼ Change IV bag to 5% normal saline or Ringer's lactate, KVO.

EMT–P LEVEL

▼ Conduct Scene Survey.

▼ Conduct Primary Assessment.

▼ Airway management should include a change to a mask with a high administration of O_2.

- Assess ECG, showing an normal sinus rhythm with multifocal PVCs.
- Check allergies to lidocaine. Administer lidocaine 1.0 to 1.5 mg/kg, IVP.
- Administer a lidocaine drip infusing 1 g at 1 to 2 mg per minute (one–half the normal infusion due to patient's liver problems.)
- Reassess ECG, airway, breathing, circulation, and level of consciousness.
- Conduct Secondary Assessment.
- Change IV bag to normal saline or Ringer's lactate, KVO. Draw blood sample.

AT THIS TIME, THE PATIENT'S ECG RHYTHM SHOWS AN NSR WITHOUT PVCs. (HE STILL COMPLAINS OF CHEST PAIN.)

- Administer nitroglyerin, SL or morphine sulfate, IV.
- Reassess ECG, airway, breathing, circulation, and level of consciousness.

AT THIS TIME, YOU BEGIN TO NOTE MORE PVCS ON THE MONITOR. THEN THE RHYTHM GOES INTO A MONOMORPHIC VENTRICULAR TACHYCARDIA AND THE PATIENT BECOMES UNCONSCIOUS (STILL WITH A PULSE AND RESPIRATIONS).

- Consider diazepam, 5.0 mg, IV, or as per local protocols, for sedation.
- Perform an unsynchronized cardioversion at 100 joules ASAP.
- Airway management should include proper application of the bag–valve–mask device with 100% O_2 administration.
    - Position patient properly.
    - Open airway with head–tilt, chin–lift.
    - Insert naso/oropharyngeal airway.
- Reassess ECG, airway, breathing, circulation, and level of consciousness.

AT THIS TIME, THE PATIENT IS APNEIC AND PULSELESS, WHILE VENTRICULAR FIBRILLATION SHOWS ON THE MONITOR.

- Defibrillate at 200 joules and reassess ECG.
- Defibrillate at 300 joules and reassess ECG.
- Defibrillate at 360 joules and reassess ECG and pulse.
- Initiate proper CPR.
    - 5 to 1 ratio of compressions to ventilations.
    - 80 to 100 compressions per minute.
    - Proper hand placement and depth of compression.
- Complete oral intubation with appropriate–sized tube.
    - Hyperventilate before and after.

- ▾ No longer than 30 seconds.
  - ▾ Assess lung sounds.
- ▾ Administer 1 mg of epinephrine, 1:10,000, IV, every 3 to 5 minutes while the patient is pulseless.
- ▾ (New ACLS guidelines suggest that higher doses of epinephrine may be administrered in lieu of low doses if these are ineffective. Local protocols should dictate the amount to be given at the next interval.)
- ▾ Defibrillate at 360 joules and reassess ECG and pulse.
- ▾ Continue CPR with constant pulse checks with and without compressions.

AT THIS TIME, THE PATIENT'S ECG REVEALS A SINUS TACHYCARDIA WITH A CORRESPONDING-PULSE (WITH NO SPONTANEOUS BREATHS).

- ▾ Reassess ECG, airway, breathing, circulation, and level of consciousness.
- ▾ Re–administer lidocaine drip infusing 1 g at 1 to 2 mg per min. and reassess.
- ▾ (The new ACLS standards do not recommend prophylactic lidocaine boluses with the return of a pulse unless PVCs are present. Local protocols should be followed.)

PATIENT'S BP = 60 BY PALPATION

- ▾ Place patient in Trendelenburg and reassess.
- ▾ Administer fluid bolus of 200 cc of Ringer's lactate or normal saline and reassess.
- ▾ Administer an infusion of dopamine, as per local protocols.

PATIENT'S BP = 90 BY PALPATION.

- ▾ Transport ASAP.
- ▾ Notify appropriate receiving facility.
- ▾ Obtain glucose level reading with a glucometer/glucostrip, since the patient has a history of alcoholism.

GLUCOSE READING = 67 MG/DL.

- ▾ Administer 50% dextrose, IV.
- ▾ Reassess airway, breathing, circulation, and level of consciousness.

ADDITIONAL PROBLEMS

Depending on the level of the candidate, the following problems can be added to the scenario:

1. During the scenario, just prior to the patient's rhythm change, have the patient vomit.

2. Any history (such as seizures) can be given initially, but the proper treatment for the history should be followed during the arrest (that is, blood drawn, proper solution administered).

3. During airway management, the endotracheal tube placement can take too long or be improperly placed in the right bronchus. It can also never be placed in the trachea, requiring the candidate to insert an esophageal airway.

4. The candidate can be taken further down each algorithm before the instructor elects to bring the patient out of ventricular tachycardia or ventricular fibrillation.

5. The patient may not truly go into ventricular fibrillation; it may only be a disconnected lead or a problem with the monitor.

6. Any location can be given to test the candidate's street and address competency using local running cards.

7. Any scene hazard can be incorporated at the presenter's discretion. (This is in addition to or replacement of those already mentioned.)

8. During the scenario, CPR is ineffective, requiring a change in compression depth.

9. After administering dopamine, the patient can begin to have ectopy on the ECG monitor.

10. Recurrent episodes of ventricular tachycardia or frequent PVCs can occur requiring other anti–dysrhyhmics.

SUMMARY

This patient, despite the fact that he had no history of heart disease, did have an irritable heart, as is indicated by the multifocal PVC's noted on the monitor. The initial treatment of this kind of dysrhythmia is lidocaine, IVP. This should depress phase 4 depolarization of the myocardium and terminate the ectopy. With this patient, though, the normal dosage of a lidocaine bolus was given, but the infusion dosage was reduced by half because of the patient's liver disease since the liver is the site of detoxification of lidocaine. The chest pain can be addressed with nitroglycerin, since this will dilate the coronary arteries and decrease the preload and afterload, thus reducing the myocardial work due to oxygen deficit seen in AMIs.

The onset of lethal dysrhythmias may be the first sign of heart disease and this patient had the typical R on T phenomenon, which results in an unstable ventricular tachycardia. In any patient who presents with unconsciousness, pulmonary edema, or hypotension, an unsynchronized cardioversion is the appropriate treatment, because the rhythm is so unstable we can not wait for the delay of the synchronizer.

Once in ventricular fibrillation, it's the rapid assessment of the rhythm, the quick defibrillations and the proper drug therapy that brings the patient around. The longer this rhythm persists, the more difficult it is to convert.

It should be noted that new studies suggest that any patient suspected of having an AMI should be given aspirin to be swallowed or chewed at 150 to 325 mg to reduce the incidence of re–infarction and consequently mortality.[3]

CARDIAC SCENARIO 6

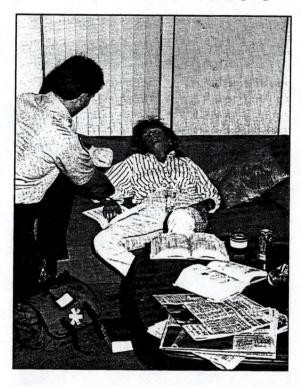

Type: Cardiac.
Scenario moulage/prop list: Live model or mannequin, grease paint for pale skin color, glycerin water for skin, pizza box (living–room setting).

[3]"Guidelines for Cardiopulmonary Resuscitation and Emergency Care," JAMA, 268 (1992), No. 16, 2170–2298.
J.E. Willard, R.A. Lange, and L.D. Hillis, "The Use of Aspirin in Ischemic Heart Disease," N. Eng J Med, 327 (1992), 175–81.

INITIAL SCENE DESCRIPTION

Dispatch Information

LOCATION: Apartment near a local college
NUMBER OF VICTIMS: 1
TYPE OF SITUATION: Dizziness
HAZARDS: None
WEATHER CONDITIONS: Clear night
TIME OF DAY: 0003 hours

Scene

You are called to the apartment of a 38–year–old, female student about midnight. She says she's been studying for exams all day and is now complaining of dizziness, shortness of breath, and a "racing heart." You immediately inquire about drug abuse as you begin to get out your equipment. She denies any drug abuse and says the only medication she takes is a birth control pill. She also says she ate some pizza about an hour ago.

Vital signs are taken and are as follows: respirations 28 and shallow, pulse too rapid to count but present radially, and BP 120/70. ECG assessment reveals this patient is in an atrial fibrillation with a rate of 160 to 170 BPM.

After placing her on O_2 via a nasal canula at 6 lpm, you establish an IV of normal saline and contact the hospital for orders. The ER physician asks you to try a few vagal maneuvers and, if unsuccessful, give 5 mg of verapamil "slow" IVP. He then tells you that if you have any problems to follow your SOP and he will see you at the emergency room.

The vagal attempts do not work and you begin to give the verapamil. As you are administering the 5 mg over 1 minute, the patient becomes extremely sluggish to respond. You discontinue the drug and begin to evaluate the patient.

PRIMARY ASSESSMENT FINDINGS

SCENE SURVEY

- ▼ apartment setting
- ▼ woman sitting on couch
- ▼ no apparent hazards

AIRWAY/CERVICAL SPINE

- ▼ airway open
- ▼ no signs of trauma
- ▼ neck veins distended

BREATHING

- ▼ 10 breaths per minute, shallow
- ▼ symmetrical chest rise
- ▼ lungs clear bilaterally

CIRCULATION/HEMORRHAGE CONTROL

- ▼ regular carotid pulse, at 44
- ▼ no radial pulse
- ▼ capillary refill delayed to 5 seconds
- ▼ no obvious external blood loss

DISABILITY

- ▼ (A, V, P, U) responsive to verbal stimuli

EXPOSE AND EXAMINE

- ▼ no obvious deformity or discoloration
- ▼ skin turgor good
- ▼ skin color pale
- ▼ skin cool and diaphoretic to touch
- ▼ weight estimated at 115 lb

SECONDARY ASSESSMENT FINDINGS

VITAL SIGNS

- ▼ respirations, 10
- ▼ pulse, 44 and regular
- ▼ blood pressure, 80/40
- ▼ ECG, a third–degree heart block

HISTORY

- ▼ as above, except for the following:
    - ▼ A   none
    - ▼ M   a birth control pill
    - ▼ P   one pack a day smoker
    - ▼ L   pizza
    - ▼ E   verapamil given by you, IVP

HEAD

- ▼ no visible trauma
- ▼ no deformity on palpation
- ▼ pupils equal and reactive, sluggish

NECK

- ▼ trachea midline
- ▼ neck veins distended
- ▼ no deformity
- ▼ no discoloration

CHEST

- ▼ no visible deformity
- ▼ no discoloration
- ▼ symmetrical chest wall movement
- ▼ lung sounds clear and equal bilaterally
- ▼ no deformity, tenderness, or crepitus on palpation

ABDOMEN

- ▼ abdomen nondistended
- ▼ soft, nontender to palpation
- ▼ no masses noted
- ▼ (if checked, bowel sounds present)
- ▼ pelvic rock stable

EXTREMITIES

- ▼ no deformity
- ▼ no discoloration
- ▼ no visible signs of trauma
- ▼ capillary refill at 5 seconds
- ▼ no distal pulses present
- ▼ skin turgor good
- ▼ skin color pale
- ▼ skin cool and diaphoretic to touch
- ▼ no tenderness, crepitus, or swelling
- ▼ movement of extremities equal

NEUROLOGICAL

- ▼ conscious, disoriented
- ▼ Glascow coma scale calculated at 13
  - ▼ eye opening to voice (3)
  - ▼ verbal response is confused (4)
  - ▼ motor response, obeys (6)

SENSORY EXAM

- ▼ no deficit in sensory or motor function

BACK

- ▼ no deformity
- ▼ no discoloration
- ▼ no trauma noted

Scenario Progression and Analysis: Once the initial treatment is done and verapamil is given, this patient goes into a symptomatic third degree heart block. After administering calcium chloride in attempt to reverse the effects of the verapamil, treatment will follow ACLS guidelines, according to its bradycardic algorithm. After a pacemaker is applied, the patient will go into a ventricular fibrillation. If ACLS guidelines are followed, this patient will improve and convert to a sinus rhythm. If not, then this patient should remain in cardiac arrest.

SUGGESTED TREATMENT

EMT–A Level

This scenario is directed for EMT–Paramedic only.

EMT–I Level

This scenario is directed for EMT–Paramedic only.

EMT–P Level

- ▾ Conduct Scene Survey.
- ▾ Conduct Primary Assessment, including rapid assessment of ECG, showing a third–degree heart block.
- ▾ Airway management should include a change to a mask with a high administration of O_2.
- ▾ Administer .5 to 1 g of calcium chloride, or as per local protocols.
- ▾ Reassess ECG, airway, breathing, circulation, and level of consciousness.

THE PATIENT LEVEL OF CONSCIOUSNESS REMAINS THE SAME. ECG STILL SHOWS A THIRD–DEGREE HEART BLOCK (WITH A RATE OF 44 BPM).

- ▾ Consider sedation and apply external pacemaker.
- ▾ Reassess ECG, airway, breathing, circulation and level of consciousness.

CAPTURE IS OBTAINED AND PATIENT'S ECG NOW SHOWS A RATE OF 70 BPM.

- ▾ Reassess ECG, airway, breathing, circulation, and level of consciousness.

PATIENT'S BP = 60 BY PALPATION.

- ▾ Administer a dopamine infusion (or epinephrine) as per local protocols.

AT THIS TIME, THE PATIENT'S ECG RHYTHM SHOWS PACER SPIKES AND NO CAPTURE AND A WAVY BASE LINE WHILE THE PATIENT APPEARS UNRESPONSIVE (APNEIC AND PULSELESS.)

- Check leads and underlying ECG rhythm. Shut off infusion.
- Reassess airway, breathing, circulation, and level of consciousness.

AT THIS TIME, PATIENT'S ECG REVEALS A COARSE V–FIB.

- Defibrillate at 200 joules and reassess ECG.
- Defibrillate at 300 joules and reassess ECG.
- Defibrillate at 360 joules and reassess ECG and pulse.
- Airway management should include proper application of the bag–valve–mask device with 100% O_2 administration.
  - Position patient properly.
  - Open airway with head–tilt, chin lift.
  - Insert naso/oropharyngeal airway.
- Initiate proper CPR.
  - 5 to 1 ratio of compressions to ventilations.
  - 80 to 100 compressions per minute.
  - Proper hand placement and depth of compression.
- Complete oral intubation with appropriate sized tube.
  - Hyperventilate before and after.
  - No longer than 30 seconds.
  - Assess lung sounds.
- Administer 1 mg of epinephrine 1:10,000, IV, every 3 to 5 minutes while patient is pulseless.
- (New ACLS guidelines suggest that higher doses of epinephrine may be administered in lieu of low doses if these are ineffective. Local protocols should dictate the amount to be given at the next interval.)
- Defibrillate at 360 joules and reassess ECG and pulse.
- Continue CPR with constant pulse checks with and without compressions.
- Administer 1.5 mg/kg lidocaine, IV.
- Defibrillate at 360 joules and reassess pulse.
- Administer 1 mg epinephrine, IV, if 3 minutes has lapsed or administer 5 mg/kg of bretylium tosylate, IV (or repeat the lidocaine bolus, 1.5 mg/kg up to 3 mg/kg).
- Defibrillate at 360 joules and reassess ECG and pulse.

AT THIS TIME, THE PATIENT'S ECG REVEALS A SINUS TACHYCARDIA WITH MULTI-FOCAL PV'S AND A CORRESPONDING PULSE (RATE OF 120 WITH NO SPONTANEOUS RESPIRATIONS).

- ▼ Reassess airway, breathing, circulation, and level of consciousness.
- ▼ Administer an infusion of 1 g of lidocaine at a rate of 2 to 4 mg/min and reassess.

PATIENT'S BP = 70/40.

- ▼ Place patient in Trendelenburg and reassess.
- ▼ Administer fluid bolus of 200 cc of Ringer's lactate or normal saline and reassess.
- ▼ Administer dopamine as per local protocols and reassess.

PATIENT'S BP = 128/70.

- ▼ Transport ASAP and conduct secondary survey.
- ▼ Notify appropriate receiving facility.

ADDITIONAL PROBLEMS

At the presenter's discretion, the following problems can be added to the scenario:

1. During the scenario, just prior to the patient's rhythm change, have the patient vomit.
2. Any history (such as diabetes) can be given initially, but the proper treatment for the history should be followed during the arrest (that is, blood drawn, 50% dextrose given).
3. During airway management, the endotracheal tube placement can take too long or be improperly placed in the right bronchus. It can also never be placed in the trachea, and thus the candidate should use an esophageal airway.
4. The candidate can be taken further down the ventricular fibrillation algorithm before the instructor elects to bring the patient out.
5. Any location can be given to test the candidate's street or address competency, using local running cards.
6. Any scene hazard can be incorporated at the presenter's discretion. (This is in addition to or replacement of those already mentioned.)
7. During the scenario, CPR is ineffective, requiring a change in compression depth.
8. After administering dopamine, the patient can begin to have ectopy on the ECG monitor.
9. The calcium choride could work and the patient could return to her initial rhythm but become unresponsive.
10. The patient could have an allergic reaction to the lidocaine and seize, requiring the administration of diazepam and another antidysrhythmic.

SUMMARY

As with any female patient of child bearing age, one important question in the history should be about method of birth control used. This patient, who is on an oral birth agent, (such as estrogen with progestogen) and who also smokes, is a prime candidate for a pulmonary embolus. A pulmonary embolism can cause the acute onset of atrial fibrillation. Signs and symptoms of a pulmonary embolism include acute shortness of breath and jugular vein distention. These symptoms can also be brought on by atrial fibrillation and can mask the primary cause of the dysrhythmia. Any paramedic should consider the acute causes of atrial fibrillation when dealing with a normally healthy individual of this age. Sudden decrease in cardiac output that is seen with acute atrial fibrillation will cause the patient to become symptomatic. The loss of atrial kick contributes to this drop in cardiac output. Usually this rhythm responds well to calcium channel blockers although the administration of calcium channel blockers can cause a variety of heart blocks as a known side effect. The paramedic should be familiar with these known dysrhythmias and be prepared to treat them as needed. The antidote of choice, for calcium channel blockers, is a calcium–containing solution (like calcium chloride), which may reverse these effects, but in this instance does not. With any patient presenting the previously described signs and symptoms, the use and/or abuse of cocaine and amphetamines must be ruled out. A thorough scene survey and direct questioning of the patient are a must to help determine this kind of history.

Atropine is now considered to be possibly harmful when used to treat a third degree heart block. The pacemaker is now considered to be the frontline therapy. If the patient's hypotension is thought to be caused by the bradycardic rate, a dopamine or an epinephrine infusion may be administered as well, depending on how severe the patient's hyptoension is. As with all interventions, local protocols and medical direction should dictate procedure.[4]

---

[4] "Guidelines for Cardiopulmonary Resuscitation and Emergency Care," JAMA, 268 (1992), No. 16, 2222.

CARDIAC SCENARIO 7

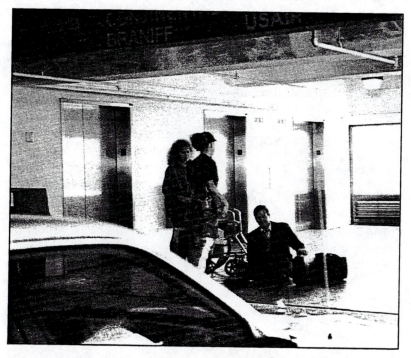

Type: Cardiac.
Scenario moulage/prop list: Live model or mannequin, small crowd, chair, suitcase, white grease paint for ashen skin color, glycerin water for skin (airport setting).

INITIAL SCENE DESCRIPTION

Dispatch Information

LOCATION: Airport terminal
NUMBER OF VICTIMS: 1
TYPE OF SITUATION: Man with chest pain
HAZARDS: None
WEATHER CONDITIONS: Sunny morning
TIME OF DAY: 0700 hours

Scene

You are dispatched to the local international airport for a man with chest pain. You arrive to find a busy airport terminal with a small crowd gathered around a

42–year–old male. The patient is complaining of severe, substernal chest pain. You note that his skin is extremely diaphoretic and cool to the touch. You also observe that his color is ashen and dusky gray. While your partner begins to administer oxygen, you question the patient. The patient states, "I just got off a flight from New York and about 1 hour ago I started to have this pressure in my chest." The patient goes on to say that the pain has been getting worse the entire time, as well as denying any shortness of breath, radiation, or nausea and vomiting. He also denies any past medical history or drug use.

PRIMARY ASSESSMENT FINDINGS

SCENE SURVEY

- international airport
- crowd of bystanders
- man sitting on floor
- no apparent hazards

AIRWAY/CERVICAL SPINE

- airway open
- no signs of trauma
- neck veins flat

BREATHING

- 20 breaths per minute, nonlabored
- symmetrical chest rise
- lungs clear bilaterally

CIRCULATION/HEMORRHAGE CONTROL

- slow, weak carotid pulse at 38
- slow, weak radial pulse at 38
- capillary refill delayed to 5 seconds
- no obvious external blood loss

DISABILITY

- (A, V, P, U) alert

EXPOSE AND EXAMINE

- no obvious deformity or discoloration
- skin color ashen and dusky gray
- skin turgor good
- skin cool and diaphoretic to touch
- weight estimated at 190 lb

SECONDARY ASSESSMENT FINDINGS

VITAL SIGNS

- ▼ respirations , 20
- ▼ pulse, 38
- ▼ blood pressure, 90/68
- ▼ ECG, a third–degree heart block

HISTORY

- ▼ as above, except for the following:
    - ▼ A   none
    - ▼ M   none
    - ▼ P   none
    - ▼ L   light meal 1 hour prior
    - ▼ E   chest pain growing more severe for 1 hour, walking

HEAD

- ▼ no visible trauma
- ▼ no deformity on palpation
- ▼ pupils equal and reactive to light

NECK

- ▼ trachea midline
- ▼ neck veins flat
- ▼ no deformity
- ▼ no discoloration

CHEST

- ▼ no visible deformity
- ▼ no discoloration
- ▼ symmetrical chest wall movement
- ▼ lung sounds clear and equal bilaterally
- ▼ no deformity, tenderness, or crepitus on palpation
- ▼ (if checked, heart sounds normal)

ABDOMEN

- ▼ abdomen nondistended
- ▼ soft, nontender to palpation
- ▼ no masses noted
- ▼ (if checked, bowel sounds present)
- ▼ pelvic rock stable

EXTREMITIES

- ▼ no deformity
- ▼ no discoloration
- ▼ no visible signs of trauma
- ▼ capillary refill delayed to 5 seconds
- ▼ slow, weak distal pulses present
- ▼ skin turgor good
- ▼ skin ashen and dusky gray
- ▼ skin cool and diaphoretic to touch
- ▼ no tenderness, crepitus, or swelling
- ▼ movement of extremities equal

NEUROLOGICAL

- ▼ conscious, alert
- ▼ Glascow coma scale calculated at 15:
    - ▼ eye opening, spontaneous (4)
    - ▼ verbal response is oriented (5)
    - ▼ motor response, obeys (6)

SENSORY EXAM

- ▼ no deficit in sensory or motor function

BACK

- ▼ no deformity
- ▼ no discoloration
- ▼ no trauma noted

Scenario Progression and Analysis: The patient's pain continues to increase in severity. As the scenario continues, the patient becomes more dyspneic. EMT As and Is should be tested on how quickly they diagnose that this is a cardiac emergency, initiate proper treatment, and transport or call for an ALS Unit. For the paramedics, the patient's level of consciousness rapidly decreases to unresponsiveness at the time of rhythm change. The patient will deteriorate from a third–degree heart block to asystole and then ventricular fibrillation. If ACLS guidelines are followed (as per American Heart Association or local protocols), the patient will improve, converting into a sinus rhythm. If they are not, the patient should remain in cardiac arrest.

SUGGESTED TREATMENT

EMT–A Level

- ▼ Conduct Scene Survey.
- ▼ Conduct Primary Assessment.

▼ Recognize the cardiac nature of this patient and transport rapidly or call for an ALS Unit.

▼ Airway management should include high–flow O_2 administration with mask.

▼ Reassess airway, breathing, circulation, and level of consciousness.

▼ Conduct Secondary Assessment.

AT THIS TIME, THE PATIENT BECOMES UNRESPONSIVE (APNEIC AND PULSELESS).

▼ Reassess airway, breathing, circulation, and level of consciousness.

▼ Airway management should include proper application of the bag–valve–mask device with 100% O_2 administration.
   ▼ Position patient properly.
   ▼ Open airway with head–tilt, chin lift.
   ▼ Insert naso/oropharyngeal airway.

▼ Initiate proper CPR.
   ▼ 5 to 1 ratio of compressions to ventilations.
   ▼ 80 to 100 compressions per minute.
   ▼ Proper hand placement and depth of compression

▼ Continue CPR while constantly assessing pulse checks with and without compressions.

▼ Transport ASAP or call for an ALS Unit, as per local protocols.

▼ Notify appropriate receiving facility.

EMT–I Level

▼ Treatment is the same as above, but includes the following:

▼ Apply automatic external defibrillator, as per local protocols.

▼ Airway management should include insertion of an esophageal airway.
   ▼ Place in sniffing position.
   ▼ Assess lung sounds.

▼ Establish a large–bore IV, infusing normal saline or Ringer's lactate KVO.

EMT–P Level:

▼ Conduct Scene Survey.

▼ Conduct Primary Assessment, which includes ECG assessment, showing a third degree heart block with a ventricular rate of 38.

▼ Airway management should include high–flow O_2 administration with mask.

▼ Establish a large–bore IV, infusing normal saline or Ringer's lactate, KVO.

▼ Administer 5 mg of valium for sedation.

- ▼ Apply external pacemaker.
- ▼ Reassess ECG, airway, breathing, circulation, and level of consciousness.

**CAPTURE IS OBTAINED. PATIENT'S ECG REVEALS
A PACED RHYTHM AT 70 BPM. PATIENT HAS
RELIEF OF CHEST PAIN. PATIENT'S BP = 120/80.**

- ▼ Conduct Secondary Assessment

**PATIENT IS NOW COMPLAINING
OF CHEST PAIN AGAIN.**

- ▼ Reassess ECG, airway, breathing, circulation, and level of consciousness.
- ▼ Administer nitroglycerin, SL or morphine sulfate, IV.
- ▼ Reassess ECG. airway, breathing, circulation, and level of consciousness.

**AT THIS TIME, THE PATIENT BECOMES UNRESPONSIVE
(APNEIC, PULSELESS WITH ASYSTOLE ON ECG).**

- ▼ Check underlying ECG rhythm and in 2 leads.
- ▼ Airway management should include proper application of the bag–valve–mask device with 100% O_2 administration.
    - ▼ Position patient properly.
    - ▼ Open airway with head–tilt, chin lift.
    - ▼ Insert naso/oropharyngeal airway.
- ▼ Initiate proper CPR.
    - ▼ 5 to 1 ratio of compressions to ventilations.
    - ▼ 80 to 100 compressions per minute.
    - ▼ Proper hand placement and depth of compression.
- ▼ Administer 1 mg of epinephrine, 1:10,000, IV, every 3 to 5 minutes while the patient is pulseless.
- ▼ Consider pacemaker again.

NO CAPTURE OBTAINED

- ▼ (New ACLS guidelines suggest that higher doses of epinephrine may be administered in lieu of low doses if these are ineffective. Local protocols should dictate the amount to be given at the next interval.)
- ▼ Reassess ECG, airway, breathing, circulation, and level of consciousness.
- ▼ Complete oral intubation with appropriate sized tube.
    - ▼ Hyperventilate before and after.
    - ▼ No longer than 30 seconds.
    - ▼ Assess lung sounds.

- Administer 1 mg of atropine, IV.
- Reassess ECG, airway, breathing, circulation, and level of consciousness.
- Continue CPR with constant pulse checks with and without compressions.

AT THIS TIME, THE ECG MONITOR SHOWS A COURSE VENTRICULAR FIBRILLATION.

- Check leads and pulse, and consider precordial thump.
- Defibrillate at 200 joules and reassess ECG.
- Defibrillate at 300 joules and reassess ECG.
- Defibrillate at 360 (or maximum) joules and reassess ECG and pulse.
- Administer 1 mg of epinephrine, 1:10,000, IV, every 3 to 5 minutes.
- Defibrillate at 360 joules and reassess ECG and pulse.
- Administer 1.5 mg/kg of lidocaine IV or ET.
- Defibrillate at 360 joules and reassess ECG and pulse.

AT THIS TIME, THE PATIENT'S ECG RHYTHM CONVERTS TO A SINUS TACHYCARDIA, RATE OF 110 BPM. (NO SPONTANEOUS RESPIRATIONS NOTED).

- Reassess ECG, airway, breathing, circulation, and level of consciousness.
- Administer a lidocaine drip infusing at 2 to 4 mg/min.
- Reassess airway, breathing, circulation, and level of consciousness.

PATIENT'S BP = 68/48.

- Place patient in trendelenburg and reassess.
- Establish another IV of Ringer's lactate or normal saline and initiate a fluid bolus of 200 cc and reasses.

PATIENT'S BP = 64/46.

- Administer dopamine as per local protocols and reassess.

PATIENT'S BP = 100/60.

- Transport ASAP.
- Notify appropriate receiving facility.
- Conduct Secondary Assessment.

ADDITIONAL PROBLEMS

Depending on the level of the candidate, the following problems can be added to the scenario:

1. During the scenario, just prior to the patient's rhythm change, have the patient vomit and lose consciousness.
2. When the candidate requests the pacemaker, do not allow its use (for instance, batteries are dead; it has been dropped and malfunctions.)
3. Any history (such as diabetes) can be given initially, but the proper treatment for the history should be followed during the arrest (that is, blood drawn, 50% dextrose given).
4. During airway management, the endotracheal tube placement can take too long or be improperly placed in the right bronchus. It can also never be placed in the trachea, requiring the candidate to use an esophageal airway.
5. The patient could return to a third-degree heart block after the last defibrillation, requiring the use of the pacemaker again.
6. IV access could be denied initially.
7. Any location can be given to test the candidate's street or address competency, using local running cards.
8. Any scene hazard can be incorporated, at the presenter's discretion. (This is in addition to or in replacement of those already mentioned).
9. Recurrent episodes of ventricular tachycardia or frequent PVCs could occur once a pulse has returned.

SUMMARY

This patient was suffering from an acute myocardial infarction to the anterior wall of the heart. Third–degree heart block is commonly seen with anterior wall infarction. Proper treatment of a third–degree heart block includes attempting to raise the ventricular rate with pacemakers with the hope of increasing the patient's perfusion.[5]

Sudden cardiac death can be the first sign of any cardiac history. It is not uncommon for patients with an acute myocardial infarction to deny any past medical history. It is important for the candidate to establish that this patient is symptomatic prior to treating this bradycardic rhythm.

As long as basic life support is being performed properly, the patient's ventilatory and circulatory status will be maintained. This alone will not convert the rhythm, but will facilitate conversion once advanced life supported is initiated.

Epinephrine is the first IV drug of choice in both the asystole and ventricular fibrillation algorithms. This and rapid defibrillations, as well as airway management, are the keys to converting ventricular fibrillation into a normal rhythm again.

---

[5]"Guidelines for Cardiopulmonary Resuscitation and Emergency Care," JAMA, 268 (1992), No. 16, 2222.

CARDIAC SCENARIO 8

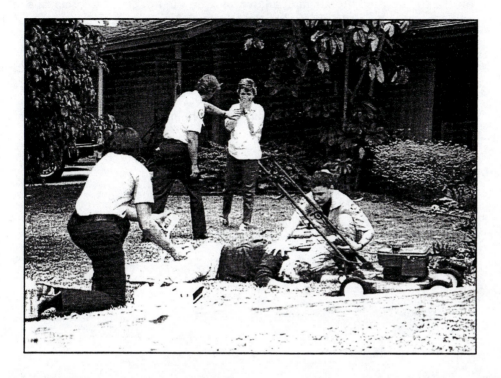

Type: Cardiac.
Scenario moulage/prop list: Live model or mannequin, live model for crying mother, outside setting, lawnmower, grease paint for cyanotic skin color, glycerin water for skin (residential home front yard setting)

INITIAL SCENE DESCRIPTION

Dispatch Information

LOCATION: Suburban home (front yard)
NUMBER OF VICTIMS: 1
TYPE OF SITUATION: Man down
HAZARDS: Running lawn mower
WEATHER CONDITIONS: Sunny day
TIME OF DAY: 1300 hours

Scene

You are en route to the scene and dispatch advises you that the woman who called is hysterical and that she cannot arouse her husband. They are unable to obtain any additional information. You arrive to find a 48–year–old male supine on the ground next to a running lawn mower. He appears unconscious, and his color is cyanotic and skin cool to the touch. The wife comes running out of the house crying loudly, stating that she could not wake him up and that he was not breathing. Your partner takes the wife to the house and begins to question her about any past medical history of the male patient. You begin a primary survey and the defibrillator arrives. The wife informs your partner that the patient does have a history of angina and one acute myocardial infarction 3 years ago. She leaves to get the names of his medications. She later states that he had no complaint prior to your arrival.

PRIMARY ASSESSMENT FINDINGS

SCENE SURVEY

- ▼ suburban home front lawn
- ▼ man lying supine in yard
- ▼ running lawnmower

AIRWAY/CERVICAL SPINE

- ▼ airway closed with tongue
- ▼ no signs of trauma
- ▼ neck veins flat

BREATHING

- ▼ no spontaneous breathing noted
- ▼ no chest rise

CIRCULATION/HEMORRHAGE CONTROL

- ▼ no carotid pulse
- ▼ no radial pulse
- ▼ capillary refill delayed and immeasurable
- ▼ no obvious external blood loss

DISABILITY

- ▼ (A, V, P, U) unresponsive

EXPOSE AND EXAMINE

- ▼ no obvious deformity or discoloration
- ▼ skin turgor good
- ▼ skin color cyanotic
- ▼ skin cool and diaphoretic to touch
- ▼ estimated weight at 200 lb

SECONDARY ASSESSMENT FINDINGS

VITAL SIGNS

- respirations, 0
- pulse, 0
- blood pressure, 0/0
- ECG, a ventricular tachycardia

HISTORY

- as above, except for the following:
    - A   none
    - M   digoxin, diltiazem, furosemide
    - P   angina, one acute myocardial infarction
    - L   light meal 1 hour prior
    - E   out cutting grass, last seen 5 minutes prior to call, found unresponsive on the lawn

HEAD

- no visible trauma
- no deformity on palpation
- pupils equal, dilated, and fixed

NECK

- trachea midline
- neck veins flat
- no deformity
- no discoloration

CHEST

- no visible deformity
- no discoloration
- symmetrical chest wall movement with respiratory support
- lung sounds clear and equal with supported ventilations
- no deformity, tenderness, or crepitus on palpation

ABDOMEN

- abdomen nondistended with no masses
- soft, nontender to palpation
- no masses noted
- (if checked, bowel sounds absent)
- pelvic rock stable

EXTREMITIES

- ▼ no deformity
- ▼ no discoloration
- ▼ no visible signs of trauma
- ▼ capillary refill delayed and immeasurable
- ▼ no distal pulses present
- ▼ skin turgor good
- ▼ skin color cyanotic
- ▼ skin cool and diaphoretic to touch
- ▼ no tenderness, crepitus, or swelling
- ▼ no movement of extremities

NEUROLOGICAL

- ▼ unconscious, unresponsive
- ▼ Glascow coma scale calculated at 3:
    - ▼ eye opening, none (1)
    - ▼ verbal response, none (1)
    - ▼ motor response, none (1)

SENSORY EXAM

- ▼ unable to determine sensory or motor function

BACK

- ▼ no deformity
- ▼ no discoloration
- ▼ no trauma noted

Scenario Progression and Analysis: This scenario begins as an unwitnessed cardiac arrest with the patient in ventricular tachycardia. EMT–As and Is should be tested on their diagnosis of a cardiac arrest, proper performance of CPR, and quickness in deciding to transport or call for an ALS Unit. For the paramedics, if proper ACLS guidelines are followed, this patient will have a rhythm change to ventricular fibrillation midway through their treatment, and then convert to an atrial fibrillation with a rate of 70 and a corresponding pulse with some spontaneous respirations. If these guidelines are not followed, this patient should remain in arrest.

SUGGESTED TREATMENT

EMT–A Level

- ▼ Conduct Scene Survey.
    - ▼ Shut off and remove mower.

- ▼ Conduct Primary Assessment.
- ▼ Recognize the cardiac nature of this patient and transport ASAP or call for an ALS Unit.
- ▼ Airway management should include proper application of the bag–valve–mask device with 100% O_2 administration.
  - ▼ Position patient properly.
  - ▼ Open airway with head–tilt, chin–lift.
  - ▼ Insert naso/oropharyngeal airway.
- ▼ Initiate proper CPR.
  - ▼ 5 to 1 ratio of compressions to ventilations.
  - ▼ 80 to 100 compressions per minute.
  - ▼ Proper hand placement and depth of compression.
- ▼ Reassess airway, breathing, circulation, and level of consciousness.
- ▼ Conduct Secondary Assessment.

EMT–I Level

- ▼ Treatment is the same as above but includes the following:
- ▼ Apply automatic external defibrillator ASAP.

THE AED DEFIBRILLATES THE PATIENT REPEATEDLY AND THEN STOPS.

- ▼ Reassess airway, breathing, circulation, and level of consciousness.

THE PATIENT IS STILL UNCONSCIOUS (BUT NOW HE HAS A CAROTID PULSE AND SPONTANEOUS BREATHS AT 4 PER MINUTE).

- ▼ Airway management should include insertion of an esophageal airway.
  - ▼ Place in sniffing position.
  - ▼ Assess lung sounds.
- ▼ Transport ASAP.
- ▼ Establish a large–bore IV, infusing normal saline or Ringer's lactate, KVO.

EMT–P Level

- ▼ Conduct Scene Survey.
  - ▼ Shut off and remove mower.
- ▼ Conduct Primary Assessment, which includes rapid ECG assessment, showing ventricular tachycardia.
- ▼ Airway management should include proper application of the bag–valve–mask device with 100% O_2 administration.

- ▼ Position patient properly.
  - ▼ Open airway with head–tilt, chin–lift.
  - ▼ Insert naso/oropharyngeal airway.
- ▼ Initiate proper CPR.
  - ▼ 5 to 1 ratio of compressions to ventilations.
  - ▼ 80 to 100 compressions per minute
  - ▼ Proper hand placement and depth of compression.
- ▼ Defibrillate at 200 joules and reassess ECG.
- ▼ Defibrillate at 300 joules and reassess ECG.
- ▼ Defibrillate at 360 (or maximum) joules and reassess ECG and pulse.
- ▼ Continue CPR.
- ▼ Complete oral intubation with appropriate–sized tube.
  - ▼ Hyperventilate before and after.
  - ▼ No longer than 30 seconds.
  - ▼ Assess lung sounds.
- ▼ Establish a large–bore IV, infusing normal saline or Ringer's lactate, KVO.
- ▼ Administer 1 mg of epinephrine, 1:10,000, IV, every 3 to 5 minutes while the patient is pulseless.
- ▼ (New ACLS guidelines suggest that higher doses of epinephrine may be administered in lieu of low doses if these are ineffective. Local protocols should dictate the amount to be given at the next interval.)
- ▼ Assess CPR constantly with pulse checks with and without compressions.
- ▼ Defibrillate at 360 joules and reassess ECG and pulse.
- ▼ Administer 1.5 mg/kg of lidocaine, IV.
- ▼ Defibrillate at 360 joules and reassess ECG and pulse.

AT THIS TIME THE PATIENT'S ECG RHYTHM CHANGES FROM VENTRICULAR TACHYCARDIA TO VENTRICULAR FIBRILLATION.

- ▼ Reassess pulse and check leads.
- ▼ Administer 1 mg of epinephrine, 1:10,000, IV, every 3 to 5 minutes while the patient is pulseless.
- ▼ Defibrillate at 360 joules and reassess ECG and pulse.
- ▼ Administer bretylium tosylate 5 mg/kg or repeat lidocaine bolus of 1.5 mg/kg up to 3 mg/kg.

AT THIS TIME, THE PATIENT'S RHYTHM SHOULD CONVERT TO AN ATRIAL FIBRILLATION (WITH A VENTRICULAR RESPONSE OF 70, A CORRESPONDING PULSE, AND SPONTANEOUS BREATHS AT 4 PER MINUTE).

- ▼ Reassess ECG, airway, breathing, circulation, and level of consciousness.
- ▼ Continue to assist with ventilations.
- ▼ Administer a lidocaine drip, infusing 2 to 4 mg/min.
- ▼ (The new ACLS standards do not recommend prophylactic lidocaine boluses with the return of a pulse unless PVCs are present. Local protocols should be followed.)

THE PATIENT'S BP = 90/58.

- ▼ Transport ASAP and conduct Secondary Assessment.
- ▼ Notify appropriate receiving facility.

AT THIS TIME, PATIENT'S ECG REVEALS MULTIFOCAL PVCS.

- ▼ Administer .5 to 1.5 mg/kg of lidocaine, IV (depending on amount of last bolus) and increase infusion.
- ▼ Reassess ECG, airway, breathing, circulation, and level of consciousness.

NO MORE PVC'S NOTED ON MONTOR.

ADDITIONAL PROBLEMS

Depending on the level of the candidate, the following problems can be added to the scenario:

1. During the scenario, make CPR ineffective and require depth change.
2. Before the defibrillator arrives, have the candidate perform one–person CPR.
3. Any history (such as diabetes) can be given initially, but the proper treatment for the history should be followed during the arrest (that is, blood drawn, 50% dextrose given).
4. During airway management, the endotracheal tube placement can take too long or be improperly placed in the right bronchus. It can also never be placed in the trachea, and thus the candidate should use an esophageal airway.
5. Following rhythm conversion to atrial fibrillation, the patient's blood pressure remains low, requiring the administration of a dopamine drip.
6. The problem of hyperthermia can be interjected, thus requiring cooling to be done once the patient is resuscitated.
7. Any location can be given to test the candidate's street or address competency, using local running cards.

8. Any scene hazard can be incorporated at the presenter's discretion. (This is in addition to or replacement of those already mentioned.)

9. Recurrent episodes of ventricular tachycardia or frequent PVCs can occur once a pulse has returned.

SUMMARY

This scenario is a standard cardiac arrest. The candidate should treat the patient as per local protocols that follow the American Heart Association ventricular fibrillation and ventricular tachycardia algorithms. Basic life support should be performed until the defibrillator arrives. As soon as the defibrillator is available, defibrillation/cardioversion should be performed. Basic life support must be performed throughout the arrest and frequently rechecked to assure adequacy.

This patient has suffered cardiac arrest from sudden cardiac death. The statistics show that many patients suffer sudden cardiac death within 2 hours of the onset of symptoms. Frequently, the first symptom is a lethal dysrhythmia without any other signs or symptoms associated. Early CPR and defibrillation have been shown to reduce out-of-hospital sudden cardiac deaths dramatically.

Chapter 2

MEDICAL SCENARIOS

MEDICAL SCENARIO 1

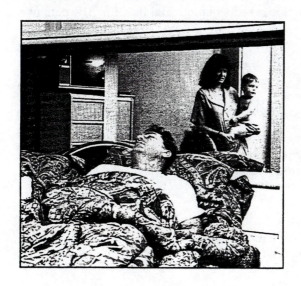

Type: Medical.
Scenario moulage/prop list: Live model or mannequin, live model for wife's role, grease paint for flushed skin color (bedroom setting with wife).

INITIAL SCENE DESCRIPTION

Dispatch Information

LOCATION: Residential house
NUMBER OF VICTIMS: 1
TYPE OF SITUATION: Shortness of breath
HAZARDS: None
WEATHER CONDITIONS: Clear, early evening
TIME OF DAY: 1835 hours

Scene

You are called to a residential house for "shortness of breath." The patient's wife greets you at the door and says her husband came home from work and has complained of shortness of breath since 1600 hours. As she walks you to the living room she explains that he seems to be getting worse. As you enter the bedroom you see a 32–year–old male in obvious respiratory distress, breathing 44 times a minute. The patient denies any history, medications, previous episodes, or any recent drug abuse. He complains of slight abdominal pain, extreme thirst, but has been unable to take fluids by mouth for the last 3 hours due to frequent vomiting that appeared to be normal in color. The patient's wife states he has not "felt right for the last 3 or 4 days." As your partner gets out a nonrebreather mask, you prepare to do a primary survey.

PRIMARY ASSESSMENT FINDINGS

SCENE SURVEY

- well-kept bedroom
- man sitting in bed
- no apparent hazards

AIRWAY/CERVICAL SPINE

- open airway
- no signs of trauma
- neck veins flat

BREATHING

- 44 breaths per minute noted, obviously labored
- symmetrical chest rise noted
- lung sounds clear bilaterally

CIRCULATION/HEMORRHAGE CONTROL

- strong carotid pulse at 112
- strong radial pulse at 112
- capillary refill delayed to 3 seconds
- no obvious external blood loss

DISABILITY

- (A, V, P, U) alert

EXPOSE AND EXAMINE

- no obvious deformity or discoloration
- skin turgor poor
- skin color flushed

- ▾ skin warm and dry to touch
- ▾ weight estimated at 210 lb

SECONDARY ASSESSMENT FINDINGS

VITAL SIGNS

- ▾ respirations, 44
- ▾ pulse, 112
- ▾ blood pressure, 90/68
- ▾ ECG, a sinus tachycardia

HISTORY

- ▾ as above, except for the following:
  - ▾ A   none
  - ▾ M   none
  - ▾ P   none
  - ▾ L   none
  - ▾ E   has not felt well for 3 or 4 days; frequent vomiting for 3 hours

HEAD

- ▾ no visible trauma
- ▾ skin flushed
- ▾ dry, cracked lips noted
- ▾ pupils equal and reactive to light

NECK

- ▾ trachea midline
- ▾ neck veins flat
- ▾ no deformity
- ▾ skin flushed

CHEST

- ▾ no visible deformity
- ▾ skin flushed on upper torso
- ▾ symmetrical chest wall movement
- ▾ lung sounds clear bilaterally
- ▾ no deformity, tenderness, or crepitus noted on palpation

ABDOMEN

- ▾ abdomen slightly distended
- ▾ soft, slightly tender to palpation
- ▾ (if checked, bowel sounds absent)
- ▾ pelvic rock stable

EXTREMITIES

- ▾ no deformity
- ▾ no discoloration
- ▾ no visible signs of trauma
- ▾ capillary refill at 3 seconds
- ▾ distal pulses present
- ▾ skin turgor poor
- ▾ skin color flushed
- ▾ skin warm and dry to touch
- ▾ no tenderness, crepitus, or swelling
- ▾ movement of extremities equal

NEUROLOGICAL

- ▾ conscious, alert
- ▾ Glasgow coma scale calculated at 15:
  - ▾ eye opening, spontaneous (4)
  - ▾ verbal response, alert (5)
  - ▾ motor response, obeys (6)

SENSORY EXAM

- ▾ no deficit in sensory or motor function

BACK

- ▾ no deformity
- ▾ no discoloration
- ▾ no trauma noted

Scenario Progression and Analysis: This patient is suffering from diabetic ketoacidosis, which explains the initial findings. The key here is to identify the signs and symptoms of DKA and not be confused by the initial complaint of shortness of breath. EMT-As and Is should be tested on proper diagnosis, airway control, and the decision to transport ASAP or call for ALS assistance. EMT-As should consider rapid transport in this particular situation and not wait for an ALS Unit. Paramedics and EMT-Is should transport ASAP, as well, and initiate an IV of Ringer's lactate since this patient is severely dehydrated. If they fail to recognize the cause of the SOB and do not transport (with volume replacement where appropriate) the patient should rapidly deteriorate into a deep coma.

SUGGESTED TREATMENT

EMT—A Level

- ▾ Conduct Scene Survey.
- ▾ Conduct Primary Assessment.

- ▼ Conduct Secondary Assessment.
- ▼ Airway management should include high–flow O_2 administration with a mask.
- ▼ Reassess airway, breathing, circulation and level of consciousness.
- ▼ Transport ASAP.
    - ▼ Do not delay for ALS Unit.
- ▼ Notify appropriate receiving facility.
- ▼ Monitor level of consciousness.

EMT-I Level

- ▼ Treatment is the same as above, but includes the following:
- ▼ Establish a large–bore IV, infusing normal saline or Ringer's lactate, as per local protocols, open.
- ▼ Reassess airway, breathing, circulation, and level of consciousness.

EMT-P Level

- ▼ Conduct Scene.
- ▼ Conduct Primary Assessment.
- ▼ Conduct Secondary.
- ▼ Airway management should include high–flow O_2 administration with a mask.
- ▼ Reassess airway, breathing, circulation, and level of consciousness.
- ▼ Draw blood sample and obtain glucometer/glucostrip reading.

GLUCOSE READING = >350 MG/DL.

- ▼ Establish a large-bore IV, infusing normal saline or Ringer's lactate, as per local protocols, open.
- ▼ Reassess airway, breathing, circulation, and level of consciousness.
- ▼ Transport ASAP.
- ▼ Notify appropriate receiving facility.
- ▼ Monitor level of consciousness.

ADDITIONAL PROBLEMS

Depending on the level of the candidate, the following problems can be added to the scenario:
1. The patient could have a seizure or become unresponsive, due to his hyperglycemia and ketoacidosis some time during the scenario.
2. The patient may lapse into coma if not rapidly diagnosed and transported.

3. The patient could vomit and aspirate, requiring vigorous suction, respiratory support, and possibly intubation.
4. Unable to obtain IV access.
5. The presenter may add any additional, underlying medical problems that he wishes to test (for example, COPD, heart disease, or hypertension).
6. Any location can be given to test the candidate's street or address competency, using local running cards.
7. Any scene hazard can be incorporated at the presenter's discretion. (This is in addition to or replacement of those already mentioned.)

SUMMARY

This scenario presents the provider with an adult–onset diabetic patient. This patient does not have any previous history of diabetes, and his chief complaint of shortness of breath is common in those who are suffering from diabetic ketoacidosis. These patients do not have sufficient levels of insulin and, without insulin, glucose cannot enter the cells to be used for energy production. Stored animal starch, called glycogen, is also released from the liver and converted into additional glucose. Consequently, this raises the levels of glucose in the bloodstream to higher than normal. The cells are still unable to utilize the increasing amount of glucose found in the blood. Eventually, the cells begin to use fats as an alternate source of energy, producing high levels of ketones as a by-product of this metabolism. These increasing levels of ketones change the Ph of the blood to a more acidic state. The body tries to reduce the acidic state in the blood by removing carbon dioxide. Carbon dioxide acts as an acid in the acid–base balance of the body and is easily removed through the lungs by increased respirations.

As the glucose level increases, the osmotic pressure begins to rise in the bloodstream. The osmotic pressure draws fluid from the interstitial and intracellular spaces. The kidneys begin to spill glucose as the level increases into the intravascular space. This spilled glucose draws fluids and electrolytes with it. The patient then begins to diurese great quantities of fluids. The amount is frequently more than can be taken in by mouth. As more fluids and electrolytes are lost, the patient begins to become dehydrated. The prehospital treatment is directed toward the ABCs first; then, as soon as possible, the provider must begin to replace the lost fluids and electrolytes. The difficulty is that the cause of the shortness of breath is often thought to be from some other source, especially in the patient with no history of diabetes.

MEDICAL SCENARIO 2

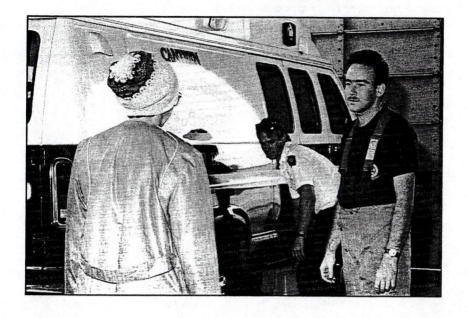

Type: Combination—medical, trauma.
Scenario moulage/prop list: Live model or mannequin, grease paint for pale skin
color, used coffee grounds around lips, rouge/grease paint to forehead for contusion, alcohol on breath, glycerin water spray bottle for skin (apparatus bay setting).

INITIAL SCENE DESCRIPTION

Dispatch Information

LOCATION: Fire Station No. 2
NUMBER OF VICTIMS: 1
TYPE OF SITUATION: Medical
HAZARDS: None
WEATHER CONDITIONS: Not pertinent
TIME OF DAY: Noon

Scene

It has been a lazy day around the station. You started lunch early when you are
notified of a "walk-in medical." You see a disheveled, elderly woman standing in
the apparatus bay. You question her as to her chief complaint, while your partner
gets the equipment from the rescue vehicle. She responds slowly, "I have been
vomiting all morning and now I am having stomach pain." You note dried cof-
fee-groundlike emesis around her mouth. She continues, saying that she has no

past medical history, although the station captain recognizes her as a local street person with "more than an occasional drinking problem."

You continue to question her because you note an old contusion of the left forehead. Still even more slowly she replies, "I fell the other day and I've had a bad headache ever since. I guess I may have had too much to drink." The patient immediately vomits a copious amount of bright, red blood and collapses unconscious to the floor.

PRIMARY ASSESSMENT FINDINGS

SCENE SURVEY

- ▼ apparatus bay
- ▼ familiar, with no hazards

AIRWAY/CERVICAL SPINE

- ▼ labored breathing complicated by bloody vomitus
- ▼ neck veins flat

BREATHING

- ▼ 8 breaths per minute, labored and shallow
- ▼ symmetrical chest rise
- ▼ lungs clear bilaterally

CIRCULATION/HEMORRHAGE CONTROL

- ▼ rapid, weak carotid pulse at 110
- ▼ no radial pulse felt
- ▼ capillary refill delayed to 8 seconds
- ▼ bright, red emesis coming from mouth
- ▼ no other external bleeding observed

DISABILITY

- ▼ (A, V, P, U) responds to painful stimuli only

EXPOSE AND EXAMINE

- ▼ old contusion left forehead
- ▼ skin turgor poor
- ▼ skin color pale
- ▼ skin cool and diaphoretic to touch
- ▼ weight estimated at 115 lb

SECONDARY ASSESSMENT FINDINGS

VITAL SIGNS

- ▼ respirations, 8
- ▼ pulse, 110

▼ blood pressure, 60/40
▼ ECG, a sinus tachycardia

HISTORY

▼ unknown, except for the following:
  ▼ A   unknown
  ▼ M   unknown
  ▼ P   alcohol abuse
  ▼ L   unknown
  ▼ E   fall a few days prior with superficial contusion
  ▼   vomiting prior to arrival
  ▼   abdominal pain

HEAD

▼ only visible deformity is to left forehead
▼ crepitus on palpation of forehead
▼ copious amount of bright, red emesis from mouth
▼ right pupil dilated and sluggishly reactive to light
▼ left pupil is midpoint and reactive to light

NECK

▼ trachea midline
▼ neck veins flat
▼ no deformity
▼ no discoloration

CHEST

▼ no visible deformity
▼ no discoloration
▼ symmetrical chest wall movement
▼ lung sounds clear and equal bilaterally
▼ no deformity, tenderness, or crepitus on palpation

ABDOMEN

▼ abdomen nondistended
▼ rigid and tender to palpation
▼ no masses noted
▼ patient moans in response to palpation
▼ (if bowel sounds checked, absent)
▼ pelvic rock stable

EXTREMITIES

▼ no deformity
▼ no discoloration

- ▾ no visible signs of trauma
- ▾ capillary refill delayed to 8 seconds
- ▾ no distal pulses present
- ▾ skin turgor poor
- ▾ skin color pale
- ▾ skin cool and diaphoretic to touch
- ▾ no tenderness, crepitus, or swelling
- ▾ equal extremity movement prior to loss of consciousness

NEUROLOGICAL

- ▾ unconscious, responds only to painful stimuli
- ▾ Glascow coma scale calculated at 7:
    - ▾ eye, opening to pain (2)
    - ▾ verbal response, none (1)
    - ▾ motor response, withdraws (4)

SENSORY EXAM

- ▾ withdraws from painful stimuli and moves all extremities appropriately

BACK

- ▾ no deformity
- ▾ no discoloration
- ▾ no trauma noted

Scenario Progression and Analysis: If both the airway and hypotension are addressed rapidly and appropriately, the patient remains the same. If either is not treated correctly, or a proper diagnosis not made and decisions to transport not rapidly accomplished, then the patient deteriorates and can go into any cardiac dysrhythmia. If BTLS/PHTLS guidelines are followed, the patient should remain the same.

SUGGESTED TREATMENT

EMT-A Level

- ▾ Conduct Scene Survey.
- ▾ Conduct Primary Assessment.
- ▾ Recognize that this is a true medical emergency and transport ASAP or call for an ALS Unit.
- ▾ Suction vigorously.
    - ▾ Hyperventilate before and after.
    - ▾ Suction only on withdrawal.

- ▾ Suction no longer than 10 seconds.
- ▾ Airway management should include proper application of the bag–valve–mask device with 100% O_2 administration.
  - ▾ Position patient properly.
  - ▾ Open airway with modified jaw thrust method.
  - ▾ Insert oropharyngeal airway.
  - ▾ Hyperventilate patient.
- ▾ Maintain cervical spine manually during and after airway management.
- ▾ Secure patient with cervical immobilization devices to backboard.
- ▾ Continue to hyperventilate patient.
- ▾ Conduct MAST survey and apply pneumatic antishock trousers, as per local protocols.
- ▾ Reassess airway, breathing, circulation, and level of consciousness.

PATIENT'S BP = 60/40.

- ▾ Consider elevation of the head of the backboard 15 degrees to help decrease intracranial pressure, once blood pressure has improved.
- ▾ Conduct secondary survey.

EMT-I Level

- ▾ Treatment is the same as above, but includes the following:
- ▾ Apply the automatic external defibrillator, as per local protocols.
- ▾ Establish at least two large–bore IVs, infusing normal saline or Ringer's lactate, as per local protocols, open.
- ▾ Reassess airway, breathing, circulation, and level of consciousness.

EMT-P Level

- ▾ Conduct Scene Survey.
- ▾ Conduct Primary Assessment, including rapid assessment of ECG, showing a sinus tachycardia.
- ▾ Suction vigorously.
  - ▾ Hyperventilate before and after.
  - ▾ Suction only on withdrawal.
  - ▾ Suction no longer than 10 seconds.
- ▾ Airway management should include proper application of the bag–valve–mask device with 100% O_2 administration.
  - ▾ Position patient properly.
  - ▾ Open airway with modified jaw thrust method.
  - ▾ Insert oropharyngeal airway.

- Maintain cervical spine manually during and after airway management.
- Secure patient with cervical immobilization devices to backboard.
- Complete oral intubation with appropriate–sized tube.
  - Hyperventilate before and after.
  - No longer than 30 seconds.
  - Assess lung sounds.
  - Continue to hyperventilate patient.
- Conduct MAST survey and apply pneumatic antishock garment, as per local protocols.
- Reassess airway, breathing, circulation, and level of consciousness.

PATIENT'S BP = 60/40.

- Consider elevation of the head of the backboard 15 degrees to help decrease intracranial pressure, once blood pressure has improved.
- Transport ASAP.
- Establish at least two large-bore IVs, infusing normal saline or Ringer's lactate, as per local protocols, open.
- Reassess airway, breathing, circulation, and level of consciousness.
- Draw blood sample and obtain glucometer/glucostrip reading due to the patient's history of alcoholism.

GLUCOSE READING = 62 MG/DL.

- Administer 50% dextrose, IV.
- Reassess airway, breathing, circulation, and level of consciousness.

PATIENT'S LEVEL OF CONSCIOUSNESS DOES NOT CHANGE.

- Administer 2 mg of naloxone, IV.
- Administer thiamine, as per local protocols.
- Conduct secondary survey.

ADDITIONAL PROBLEMS

Depending on the level of the candidate, the following problems can be added to the scenario:

1. If universal precautions are not followed, the candidate can be told, after the scenario, that the patient had HIV or hepatitis.
2. The patient can go into any cardiac dysrhythmia that you wish to test.
3. If suctioning is carried out for too great a period of time, the patient can develop ectopic beats and/or dysrhythmias.
4. If the esophageal airway is used, the patient should deteriorate and become pulseless.

5. The patient can seize, even if the head injury is properly addressed, requiring intervention with diazepam.
6. After 50% dextrose is given, all IV lines can infiltrate, requiring that all other drugs be given ET.
7. After IV lines have been established, the patient can deteriorate and go into cardiac arrest to further test the candidate's knowledge.
8. Any location can be given to test the candidate's street or address competency, using local running cards.
9. Any scene hazard can be incorporated at the presenter's discretion. (This is in addition to or replacement of those already mentioned.)

SUMMARY

This woman was a chronic alcoholic. Seizures, esophageal varices, and head injuries are common problems associated with this type of patient. The fall several days prior created a slow, subdural bleed. As a result of years of alcohol abuse, esophageal varices had formed; these ruptured, causing a massive hemorrhage, leading to her hypovolemia. Alcohol use can complicate the patient assessment and make obtaining a history difficult.

Proper treatment includes cervical spine immobilization, effective airway control and oxygenation, proper volume infusion, and rapid transport to an appropriate receiving facility. In any unconscious alcoholic, 50% dextrose and naloxone should be considered to reverse any hypoglycemia or narcotic overdose. Thiamine should be also be considered to prevent Wernicke's encephalopathy, which is sometimes seen in alcoholics.

This patient should be hyperventilated, and elevation of the head of the backboard by 15 degrees should be considered to reduce the patient's cerebral swelling, if the hypotension improves. Esophageal airways are contraindicated in any patient with possible esophageal bleeding. For this scenario, airway management with nasal adjuncts and/or intubation was also avoided, by the authors, due to the possibility of a skull fracture. Many physicians feel that nasal intubation can be used in the absence of facial trauma for airway control. Since this text is meant for national consumption, the authors chose to avoid this particular intervention since the degree of injury cannot be determined in the absence of diagnostic X-rays. Local protocols should address proper management in this area.

Medical direction has suggested that the administration of furosemide is beneficial for the management of increased intracranial pressure. Furosemide has been proven to reduce cerebral edema in head injury patients. The authors recognize that in this scenario, as presented, the patient is hypotensive and this may preclude its administration. But, depending on local protocols, it should be considered.[6]

6"Guidelines for Cardiopulmonary Resuscitation and Emergency Care," JAMA, 268 (1992), No. 16, 2171–2298.
    Patricia A. Tornheim, "Effect of Furosemide on Experimental Traumatic Cerebral Edema," Neurosurgery 4 (1979) No. 1, 48–52.

MEDICAL SCENARIO 3

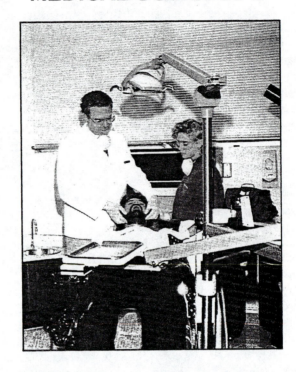

Type: Medical—combination of anaphylaxis and diabetes.
Scenario moulage/prop list: Live model or mannequin, live model dressed as dentist, nasal canula, grease paint for pale skin color, glycerin water for skin (dental office setting).

INITIAL SCENE DESCRIPTION

Dispatch Information

LOCATION: Dentist office
NUMBER OF VICTIMS: 1
TYPE OF SITUATION: Possible respiratory arrest
HAZARDS: None
WEATHER CONDITIONS: Cloudy morning
TIME OF DAY: 0815 hours

Scene

You just begin to check out your truck when the first call of the day interrupts you. En route, you are told that this is a medical alarm at a dentist's office and that a dental hygienist just called back to say that the patient is a diabetic and in respiratory arrest. You arrive at the office to find both the dentist and his staff in a frantic state. Upon evaluation of the patient, you find a 35–year–old male sitting up in a dental chair, who in fact is not in respiratory arrest, but is obviously in acute respiratory distress (so much that he cannot utter a word), breathing 44 times a minute with expiratory wheezes that can be heard from across the room. A nasal canula is in place at 2 lpm.

The dentist explains that he was preparing the patient for a tooth extraction, and after he injected a local anesthetic, the patient began to become short of breath. He quickly goes over the patient's chart and you find out that he is a new patient who stated that he had no allergies, but had a history of being an insulin-dependent diabetic, and was instructed "not to eat anything that morning."

The patient is responsive to verbal stimuli and his skin is cool and diaphoretic.

PRIMARY ASSESSMENT FINDINGS

SCENE SURVEY

- dentist office with man in chair
- no apparent hazards

AIRWAY/CERVICAL SPINE

- airway open
- no signs of trauma
- neck veins flat
- edema noted to neck

BREATHING

- 44 breaths per minute, severely labored
- symmetrical chest rise
- audible expiratory wheezes

CIRCULATION/HEMORRHAGE CONTROL

- regular, rapid carotid pulse at 120
- regular, rapid radial pulse at 120
- capillary refill at 3 seconds
- no obvious external blood loss

DISABILITY

- (A, V, P, U) responsive to verbal stimuli

EXPOSE AND EXAMINE

- rash and hives to chest and neck
- skin turgor good
- skin color pale

- ▼ skin cool and diaphoretic to touch
- ▼ weight estimated at 180 lb

SECONDARY ASSESSMENT FINDINGS

VITAL SIGNS

- ▼ respirations, 44 and labored
- ▼ pulse, 120 and regular
- ▼ blood pressure, 90/60
- ▼ ECG, a sinus tachycardia

HISTORY

- ▼ as above, except for the following:
  - ▼ A   no previous history of allergies
  - ▼ M   insulin
  - ▼ P   diabetes
  - ▼ L   none
  - ▼ E   given a local anesthetic by the dentist

HEAD

- ▼ no visible trauma
- ▼ no deformity on palpation
- ▼ pupils equal and reactive, sluggish

NECK

- ▼ trachea midline
- ▼ neck veins flat
- ▼ edema noted to neck
- ▼ hives noted on right side of neck

CHEST

- ▼ rash and hives noted on upper chest
- ▼ symmetrical chest wall movement
- ▼ lung sounds wheezing, all fields
- ▼ no tenderness or crepitus on palpation

ABDOMEN

- ▼ abdomen nondistended
- ▼ soft, nontender to palpation
- ▼ (if checked, bowel sounds present)
- ▼ pelvic rock stable

EXTREMITIES

- ▼ no deformity
- ▼ no discoloration
- ▼ no visible signs of trauma

- capillary refill at 3 seconds
- distal pulses present
- skin turgor good
- skin pale
- skin cool and diaphoretic to touch
- no tenderness, crepitus, or swelling
- movement of extremities equal

NEUROLOGICAL

- conscious, only opens eyes to voice
- Glascow coma scale calculated at 14:
    - eye, opening to voice (3)
    - verbal response, unable to speak due to respiratory status (5)
    - motor response, obeys (6)

SENSORY EXAM

- no deficit in sensory or motor function

BACK

- no deformity
- no discoloration
- no trauma noted

Scenario Progression and Analysis: This patient is both hypoglycemic, due to his lack of eating, and suffering from anaphylaxis due to the local anesthetic injection. EMT-As and Is should be tested on how quickly they diagnose the problems, initiate the proper treatment, and transport or call for ALS assistance. Paramedics should be tested on how quickly they diagnose the problems, administer the epinephrine subcutaneously, and treat the hypoglycemia. Treatment for the anaphylaxis should be done first, followed by the treatment for hypoglycemia. If the diagnosis and treatment are completed rapidly, the patient's respirations will slow to within normal limits and the wheezing will subside. The patient will also become more alert after the 50% Dextrose. If this treatment is not accomplished, the patient should go into respiratory arrest followed by cardiac arrest.

SUGGESTED TREATMENT

EMT-A Level

- Conduct Scene Survey.
- Conduct Primary Assessment.
- Recognize this as a true respiratory emergency and transport rapidly or call for an ALS Unit.
- Airway management should include a change to a mask with a high admin-

istration of O_2

- ▼ Reassess airway, breathing, circulation, and level of consciousness.
- ▼ Notify appropriate receiving facility.
- ▼ Administer glucogel, by mouth or as per local protocols.
- ▼ Conduct Secondary Assessment.

EMT-I Level

- ▼ Treatment is the same as above, but includes the following:
- ▼ Establish a large-bore IV infusing normal saline, as per local protocols, KVO.

EMT-P Level

- ▼ Conduct Scene Survey.
- ▼ Conduct Primary Assessment.
- ▼ Airway management should include a change to a mask with a high administration of O_2
- ▼ Complete assessment of ECG rhythm, showing a sinus tachycardia without ectopy.
- ▼ Establish an IV, infusing normal saline, as per local protocols, KVO.
- ▼ Administer 0.3 to .5 mg of epinephrine, 1 : 1000, subcutaneously.
- ▼ Reassess ECG, airway, breathing, circulation, and level of consciousness.

AT THIS TIME, THE PATIENT'S BREATHING BEGINS TO SLOW DOWN AND THE LUNGS ARE FOUND TO BE CLEAR. PATIENT IS STILL RESPONSIVE ONLY TO VOICE.

- ▼ Administer 50 mg of diphenhydramine, IV.
- ▼ Reassess ECG, airway, breathing, circulation and level of consciousness.
- ▼ Draw blood sample and obtain glucometer/glucostrip reading.

GLUCOSE READING = 17 MG/DL.

- ▼ Administer 50% dextrose, IV.
- ▼ Reassess ECG, airway, breathing, circulation, and level of consciousness.

AT THIS TIME, THE PATIENT BECOMES ALERT.

- ▼ Transport ASAP.
- ▼ Conduct Secondary Assessment.
- ▼ Notify appropriate receiving facility.

ADDITIONAL PROBLEMS

Depending on the level of the candidate, the following problems can be added to the scenario:

1. The patient's wheezing can continue so that the candidate should administer another epinephrine, 1 : 1000, subcutaneously.

2. Due to the anaphylaxis, the patient can go into respiratory arrest and have to be intubated.

3. The patient can then have a complete airway obstruction, requiring a cricothyrotomy or transtracheal jet insufflation to make the airway patent.

4. The hypoglycemia reading can remain low, even after the initial administration of 50% dextrose, requiring the candidate to administer another ampule.

5. Any scene hazard can be incorporated at the presenter's discretion. (This is in addition to or replacement of those already mentioned.)

6. After the proper treatment has been accomplished, the patient can still deteriorate and go into cardiac arrest to further test the candidate's knowledge.

7. Any location can be given to test the candidate's street or address competency, using local running cards.

SUMMARY

A common setting for many of the allergic reactions a prehospital care provider will encounter may be a dentist's office. The combination of the administration of local anesthetics and the fact that some dentists are not equipped to handle any kind of emergency makes these calls particularly challenging. An allergic reaction of this type is the result of several different factors: One is that the lidocaine used for cardiac administration does not have preservatives, while the lidocaine used for local anesthesia does contain certain preservatives that patients can react to. The second factor is that local anesthetics contain a small dose of epinephrine to reduce bleeding and prolong the effects of the drug, thus mimicking a reaction. Any kind of shock or physiological insult can precipitate hypoglycemia in the diabetic patient. The anaphylaxis increases the cellular demand for glucose and could cause hypoglycemia in the insulin-dependent diabetic.

The treatment for anaphylaxis is directed toward the reversal of bronchoconstriction and improved ventilation and oxygenation. The effects of epinephrine will also reverse vasodilation and the loss of vascular tone that occurs in anaphylaxis. The allergic reaction is caused by a release of substances from mast cells and basophils. Histamine and heparin are two of these. A variety of symptoms are caused by these substances, some of which can be reversed by an antihistamine such as diphenhydramine.

MEDICAL SCENARIO 4

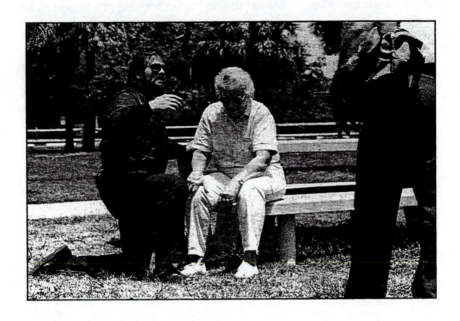

Type: Medical, anaphylaxis.
Scenario moulage/prop list: Live model or mannequin, live model for ranger's role, grease paint for hives and rash skin color, glycerin water for skin (picnic area setting).

INITIAL SCENE DESCRIPTION

Dispatch Information

LOCATION: Picnic area
NUMBER OF VICTIMS: 1
TYPE OF SITUATION: Possible allergic reaction
HAZARDS: None
WEATHER CONDITIONS: Sunny morning
TIME OF DAY: 1015 hours

Scene

You are dispatched to a local park for an "allergic reaction." You are directed to the picnic area by dispatch, where you find a 68-year-old female in the care of a park ranger. He states that the woman was stung by an insect 5 minutes prior to his calling of 911. Her original complaint was swelling of the lips and tongue. As you begin to question her you note the swelling of these areas. She is now complaining of difficulty breathing.

PRIMARY ASSESSMENT FINDINGS

SCENE SURVEY

- picnic area with woman sitting leaning forward on table
- no apparent hazards

AIRWAY/CERVICAL SPINE

- swelling noted in lips and tongue
- no signs of trauma
- neck veins flat

BREATHING

- 26 breaths per minute, shallow and labored
- symmetrical chest rise
- lung sounds reveal inspiratory wheezes bilaterally

CIRCULATION/HEMORRHAGE CONTROL

- weak, rapid carotid pulse at 116
- weak, rapid radial pulse at 116
- capillary refill delayed to 4 seconds
- no obvious external blood loss

DISABILITY

- (A, V, P, U) alert

EXPOSE AND EXAMINE

- skin color flushed with raised, reddened rash noted on left upper arm, shoulder, chest, and neck
- skin turgor good
- skin warm and diaphoretic to touch
- weight estimated at 140 lb

SECONDARY ASSESSMENT FINDINGS

VITAL SIGNS

- respirations, 26
- pulse, 116 and regular
- blood pressure, 88/50
- ECG, a sinus tachycardia

HISTORY

▼ as above, except for the following:
- ▼ A   bee stings
- ▼ M   nitro-dur, bee sting kit
- ▼ P   angina
- ▼ L   fried chicken 1 hour before
- ▼ E   the patient says she was stung by an insect and then self-administered epinephrine 0.3 mg, subcutaneously, via an autoinjector to her left thigh (time elapsed 6 minutes)

HEAD

- ▼ no visible trauma
- ▼ continued swelling to lips and tongue
- ▼ no deformity on palpation
- ▼ pupils dilated and reactive, sluggish

NECK

- ▼ trachea midline
- ▼ neck veins flat
- ▼ rash noted on left side of neck
- ▼ insect bite on left side of neck

CHEST

- ▼ no visible trauma
- ▼ rash visibly noted on left shoulder, chest
- ▼ symmetrical chest wall movement
- ▼ nitro-dur patch noted right anterior chest
- ▼ lung sounds wheezing, all fields
- ▼ no deformity, tenderness, or crepitus on palpation

ABDOMEN

- ▼ abdomen nondistended
- ▼ soft, nontender to palpation
- ▼ (if checked, bowel sounds present)
- ▼ pelvic rock stable

EXTREMITIES

- ▼ no deformity
- ▼ rash to left arm
- ▼ no visible signs of trauma
- ▼ capillary refill 4 seconds

- weak, distal pulses present
- skin turgor good
- skin color flushed
- skin warm and diaphoretic to touch
- no tenderness or crepitus
- swelling feet noted
- movement of extremities equal

NEUROLOGICAL

- conscious, alert
- Glascow coma scale calculated at 15:
    - Eye opening to voice (4)
    - verbal response, unable to speak due to respiratory status (5)
    - motor response, obeys (6)

SENSORY EXAM

- no deficit in sensory or motor function

BACK

- no deformity
- rash noted on entire back and buttocks
- no trauma noted

Scenario Progression and Analysis: This patient is both hypotensive and in acute respiratory distress due to anaphylaxis following a bee sting. EMT-As and Is should be tested on how quickly they diagnose the problem, initiate the proper treatment, and transport or call for ALS assistance. Paramedics should be tested on how quickly they diagnose the problems, readminister the epinephrine subcutaneously, reevaluate the patient, and treat the hypotension. This patient will remain slightly hypotensive until she receives a fluid bolus. All should remove the nitro–dur patch once patient is found to be hypotensive. If the diagnosis and treatment are completed rapidly, the patient's respirations will slow to within normal limits and the wheezing will subside. If this treatment is not accomplished, the patient should go into respiratory arrest and then cardiac arrest.

SUGGESTED TREATMENT

EMT-A Level

- Conduct Scene Survey.
- Conduct Primary Assessment.
- Recognize this as a true respiratory emergency and transport rapidly or call for an ALS Unit.

- ▼ Airway management should include high–flow O_2 administration with a mask.
- ▼ Reassess airway, breathing, circulation and level of consciousness.
- ▼ Notify appropriate receiving facility.
- ▼ Conduct Secondary Assessment.
- ▼ Remove nitro-dur patch.

EMT-I Level

- ▼ Treatment is the same as above, but includes the following:
- ▼ Establish a large–bore IV infusing normal saline, as per local protocols, open.
- ▼ Reassess airway, breathing, circulation, and level of consciousness.

EMT-P Level

- ▼ Conduct Scene Survey.
- ▼ Conduct Primary Assessment.
- ▼ Airway management should include high–flow O_2 administration with a mask.
- ▼ Complete assessment of ECG rhythm, showing a sinus tachycardia without ectopy.
- ▼ Establish a large-bore IV, infusing normal saline, as per local protocols, KVO.
- ▼ Readminister 0.3 to .5 mg of epinephrine, 1 : 1000, subcutaneously.
- ▼ Reassess ECG, airway, breathing, circulation, and level of consciousness.

AT THIS TIME, THE PATIENT'S BREATHING BEGINS TO SLOW DOWN AND THE LUNGS ARE FOUND TO BE CLEAR.

- ▼ Administer 50 mg of diphenhydramine, IV.
- ▼ Reassess ECG, airway, breathing, circulation and level of consciousness.
- ▼ Conduct Secondary Assessment.
- ▼ Remove nitro-dur patch.

PATIENT'S BP = 88/50.

- ▼ Administer fluid bolus of 200 cc of Ringer's lactate or normal saline.
- ▼ Reassess ECG, airway, breathing, circulation and level of consciousness.

PATIENT'S BP = 104/56.

ECG = SINUS TACHYCARDIA WITH PVC COUPLETS.

▾ Check allergies to lidocaine. Administer 1–1.5 mg/kg of lidocaine, IV, followed by a drip of 1 g of lidocaine, infusing at a rate of 2 to 4 mg/min.
▾ Reassess ECG, airway, breathing, circulation, and level of consciousness.

ECG = SINUS TACHYCARDIA WITH NO MORE PVCS.

▾ Transport ASAP.
▾ Notify appropriate receiving facility.

ADDITIONAL PROBLEMS

Depending on the level of the candidate, the following problems can be added to the scenario:

1. The patient can continue to have PVCs, even after the initial bolus and drip, requiring additional interaction with more lidocaine.
2. Due to the anaphylaxis, the patient can go into respiratory arrest, requiring intubation.
3. The patient can have a complete airway obstruction, requiring a cricothyrotomy or transtracheal jet insufflation.
4. The patient's BP can remain low or become even lower, requiring additional boluses or application of the pneumatic antishock garment.
5. Any scene hazard can be incorporated at the presenter's discretion. (This is in addition to or replacement of those already mentioned.)
6. Even after the proper treatment has been accomplished, the patient can still deteriorate and go into cardiac arrest to further test the candidate's knowledge.
7. The presenter may add any additional, underlying medical problems that he or she wishes to test (for example, COPD, heart disease, or hypertension).
8. After the nitro-dur patch is removed and the patient's hypotension and ectopy are addressed, the patient can begin to complain of chest pain.
9. Any location can be given to test the candidate's street or address competency, using local running cards.
10. The patient could have a medical alert bracelet with allergies to "Novacain," requiring the use of another antidysrhythmic for the PVCs.

SUMMARY

As with all anaphylaxis emergencies, the prehospital care provider should focus on the ABCs initially. The release of substances, including histamine and heparin, by mast cells and basophils leads to bronchial constriction, vasodilation, and capillary sieving. The results are profound respiratory distress because of the bronchial constriction. Vasodilation and capillary sieving lead to hypotension and hypovolemia. Epinephrine reduces the bronchial constriction and counteracts the vascular dilation through its alpha/beta effects. Diphenhydramine prevents any further effects of histamine release by blocking its effects at the histamine receptor sites.

Self-administration of epinephrine is becoming more frequent with the introduction of autojet administration sets. The prehospital care provider should be familiar with the dosage of these devices. Repeated doses of epinephrine may be required for the anaphylactic patient. The administration of epinephrine can precipitate cardiac dysrhythmias, but this is uncommon and rarely causes a problem. In any patient over 40 years of age, caution should be taken to observe and treat any cardiac dysrhythmias

MEDICAL SCENARIO 5

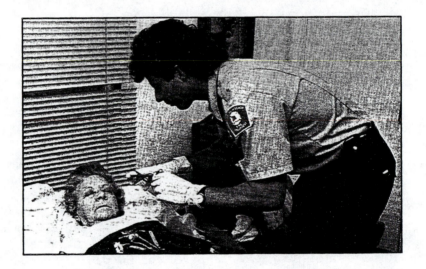

Type: Medical—CVA.
Scenario moulage/prop list: Live model or mannequin, live model for sister's role, grease paint for mottled skin color, soiled bed clothes, bed, tape of barking dog, pill bottles marked with medication names, glycerin water for skin (small bedroom setting).

INITIAL SCENE DESCRIPTION

Dispatch Information

LOCATION: Suburban single-family home
NUMBER OF VICTIMS: 1
TYPE OF SITUATION: Woman down
HAZARDS: Large barking dog chained in backyard
WEATHER CONDITIONS: Foggy, cool morning
TIME OF DAY: 0630 hours

Scene

The sister of the patient meets you at the door. She states, "I have been unable to get my sister out of the bed this morning." You enter the small, back bedroom to find a 78-year-old female with loud, snoring respirations. You attempt to arouse the patient, but she does not respond. The sister says that they went to bed last night, as usual, around 10 P.M. and that her sister had no complaints at that time. The room is cool, but not uncomfortable. The patient is dressed in her bed clothes and they appear to be soiled with urine and feces.

PRIMARY ASSESSMENT FINDINGS

SCENE SURVEY

- small cramped bedroom
- woman lying supine in bed
- no apparent hazards

AIRWAY/CERVICAL SPINE

- airway partially obstructed by the tongue
- no signs of trauma
- neck veins flat

BREATHING

- 36 breaths per minute, labored and snoring respirations
- symmetrical chest rise
- lung sounds clear bilaterally

CIRCULATION/HEMORRHAGE CONTROL

- irregular, carotid pulse at 60
- irregular, radial pulse at 60
- capillary refill at 3 seconds
- no obvious external blood loss

DISABILITY

- (A, V, P, U) responsive to painful stimuli

EXPOSE AND EXAMINE

- no obvious deformity or discoloration
- skin turgor fair
- skin color mottled

- skin cool and diaphoretic to touch
- weight estimated at 140 lb

SECONDARY ASSESSMENT FINDINGS

VITAL SIGNS

- respirations, 36 snoring
- pulse, 60 and irregular
- blood pressure, 198/78
- ECG, an atrial fibrillation

HISTORY

- as above, except for the following:
    - A   penicillin
    - M   dipyridamole, lanoxin, monopril, warfrin
    - P   numerous previous TIAs, cardiac, cataract surgery on right eye
    - L   full dinner last night at 6:30 P.M.
    - E   last seen before bed last night

HEAD

- no visible trauma
- no deformity on palpation
- left pupil midpoint and reactive, sluggish
- right pupil fixed and dilated
- severe jaw tetany

NECK

- trachea midline
- neck veins flat
- no deformity
- no discoloration

CHEST

- no visible deformity
- no discoloration
- symmetrical chest wall movement
- lung sounds clear and equal bilaterally
- no deformity, tenderness, or crepitus on palpation

ABDOMEN

- abdomen nondistended
- soft, nontender to palpation

▼ (if checked, bowel sounds present)
▼ pelvic rock stable
▼ smell of urine and feces

EXTREMITIES

▼ no deformity
▼ no discoloration
▼ no visible signs of trauma
▼ capillary refill 3 seconds
▼ distal pulses present
▼ skin turgor fair
▼ skin color mottled
▼ skin cool and diaphoretic to touch
▼ no tenderness, crepitus, or swelling
▼ bilateral decerebrate posturing with no spontaneous movements

NEUROLOGICAL

▼ unconscious, decerebrate posturing in response to painful stimuli
▼ Glascow coma scale calculated at 4:
    ▼ eye opening, none (1)
    ▼ verbal response, none (1)
    ▼ motor response, decerebrate posturing (2)

SENSORY EXAM

▼ no appropriate response to painful stimuli

BACK

▼ no deformity
▼ no discoloration
▼ no trauma noted

Scenario Progression and Analysis: This patient is suffering from a CVA. EMT-A's and Is should be tested on how quickly they diagnose the problem, initiate the proper treatment, and transport or call for ALS assistance. Paramedics should be tested on how quickly they diagnose the problem, properly control the airway with nasal intubation, hyperventilate, and treat for a coma of unknown origin. Midway through the scenario, this patient will begin to have a grand mal seizure, which should be treated with diazepam. If the diagnosis and treatment are completed rapidly, the patient will remain the same. If this treatment is not accomplished, the patient should develop status epilepticus and eventually go into cardiac arrest.

SUGGESTED TREATMENT

EMT-A Level

- ▼ Conduct Scene Survey.
- ▼ Conduct Primary Assessment.
- ▼ Airway management should include proper application of the bag-valve-mask device with 100% O_2 administration.
    - ▼ Position patient properly.
    - ▼ Open airway with head-tilt, chin-lift.
    - ▼ Insert naso/oropharyngeal airway.
    - ▼ Hyperventilate patient.

(UNABLE TO INSERT OROPHARYNGEAL AIRWAY DUE TO PATIENT'S JAW TETANY.)

- ▼ Insert nasopharyngeal airway.
- ▼ Hyperventilate patient.
- ▼ Elevate patient's head 15 degrees.
- ▼ Reassess airway, breathing, circulation, and level of consciousness.
- ▼ Transport ASAP or call for an ALS Unit.
- ▼ Conduct Secondary Assessment.
- ▼ Notify appropriate receiving facility.

EMT-I Level

- ▼ Treatment is the same as above, but includes the following:
- ▼ Apply the automatic external defibrillator, as per local protocols.
- ▼ Establish a large-bore IV of normal saline, as per local protocols, KVO.

EMT-P Level

- ▼ Conduct Scene Survey.
- ▼ Conduct Primary Assessment, which includes rapid assessment of ECG, showing an atrial fibrillation.
- ▼ Airway management should include proper application of the bag-valve-mask device with 100% O_2 administration.
    - ▼ Position patient properly.
    - ▼ Open airway with head-tilt, chin-lift.
- ▼ Insert oropharyngeal airway or complete oral intubation with appropriate-sized tube.

(UNABLE TO INSERT OROPHARYNGEAL AIRWAY OR PERFORM ORAL INTUBATION DUE TO PATIENT'S JAW TETANY.)

- ▾ Hyperventilate patient.
- ▾ Nasally intubate patient with appropriate–sized tube.
  - ▾ Lubricate tube, insert right nares.
  - ▾ Listen for air movement through tube.
  - ▾ Assess lung sounds.
  - ▾ Continue to hyperventilate patient.
- ▾ Elevate patient's head 15 degrees.
- ▾ Reassess airway, breathing, circulation, and level of consciousness.
- ▾ Conduct Secondary Assessment.
- ▾ Establish a large-bore IV, infusing normal saline, as per local protocols, KVO.
- ▾ Draw blood sample and obtain glucometer/glucostrip reading.

GLUCOSE READING = 100 MG/DL.

AT THIS TIME, THE PATIENT HAS
A GRAND MAL SEIZURE.

- ▾ Continue to hyperventilate patient.
- ▾ Administer 2.5 to 5 mg of diazepam or as per local protocols.

THE PATIENT STOPS SEIZING.

- ▾ Reassess airway, breathing, circulation, and level of consciousness.
- ▾ Consider administration of naloxone, as per local protocols.
- ▾ Consider furosemide, IV, as per local protocols.
- ▾ Transport ASAP, continually assessing neurological status.
- ▾ Notify appropriate receiving facility.

ADDITIONAL PROBLEMS

Depending on the level of the candidate, the following problems can be added to the scenario:
1. Even though the history is directed toward CVA, the patient could respond to treatment for coma of unknown origin because of narcotics or hypoglycemia.
2. If an oropharyngeal airway is not in place during the seizure, the patient can obstruct the ET tube during the seizure. (This problem depends on whether or not oral intubation has been allowed.)
3. The patient can develop status epilepticus.
4. Any scene hazard can be incorporated at the presenter's discretion. (This is in addition to or replacement of those already mentioned.)
5. Even after the proper treatment has been accomplished, the patient can still deteriorate and go into cardiac arrest to further test the candidate's knowledge.

6. The presenter may add any additional, underlying medical problems that he or she wishes to test (for example, COPD, diabetes, or epilepsy).

7. Any location can be given to test the candidate's street or address competency, using local running cards.

8. When diazepam is administered, the patient can go into respiratory arrest.

9. If universal precautions are not followed, the candidate can be told, after the scenario, that the patient had HIV or hepatitis.

SUMMARY

This patient presents with the common symptoms of an intracranial hemorrhage. Since the cranium is closed when CVAs occur this will usually lead to increased intracranial pressure. The candidate should recognize the signs and symptoms of increased intracranial pressure and treat vigorously. Hyperventilation reduces the cerebral $PaCO_2$. In cerebral circulation, CO_2 and acidosis cause vasodilation and an increase in perfusion pressure. By reducing the $PaCO_2$, the vasodilation should be reversed. This should decrease intracranial pressure (ICP), at least temporarily. The elevation of the head will further relieve increased ICP by reducing venous return to the cranial vault. The ICP can precipitate seizure activity in patients with no history of seizures. The candidate should be prepared for this early on in the scenario. Because of the possibility of drug use or hypoglycemia, the candidate should consider treatment for "a coma of unknown origin," or as per local protocols.

Medical direction has suggested that the administration of furosemide is useful for the management of increased intracranial pressure. Although not commonly used for prehospital CVAs, furosemide has been proven to be effective in reducing cerebral edema.

MEDICAL SCENARIO 6

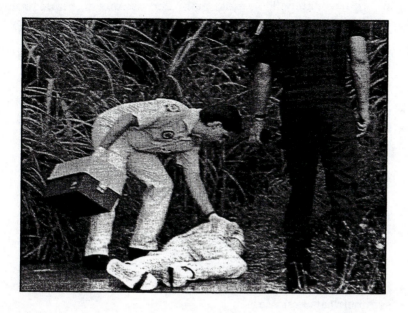

Type: combination—medical, environmental.
Scenario moulage/prop list: Live model or mannequin, live model for foreman's role, grease paint for flushed skin color, glycerin water in spray bottle for skin (agricultural field setting).

INITIAL SCENE DESCRIPTION

Dispatch Information

LOCATION: Sugarcane field
NUMBER OF VICTIMS: 1
TYPE OF SITUATION: Man down
HAZARDS: None
WEATHER CONDITIONS: Hot, humid morning
TIME OF DAY: 1130 hours

Scene

You are called to a sugarcane field, west of town, to the scene of a man down. The foreman meets you, as you drive up, saying that the only way that you can get to the patient is if he rides with you. While en route, he explains what happened. He says that one of the migrant workers "had a late night last night, but showed up for work this morning." He goes on to say that he was complaining of dizziness and leg cramps while in the fields earlier this morning. But when the foreman came back, the worker was having what appeared to be a seizure. He is now unconscious in the same field. Finally, you arrive at the scene, where you find an approximately 30-year-old male, unconscious and unresponsive, lying prone in the dirt. You cannot arouse him and his skin feels hot, yet dry.

PRIMARY ASSESSMENT FINDINGS

SCENE SURVEY

- ▼ sugarcane field
- ▼ man prone on ground
- ▼ no apparent hazards

AIRWAY/CERVICAL SPINE

- ▼ airway partially open
- ▼ no signs of trauma
- ▼ neck veins flat

BREATHING

- ▼ 30 breaths per minute, snoring respirations
- ▼ symmetrical chest rise
- ▼ lung sounds clear bilaterally

CIRCULATION/HEMORRHAGE CONTROL

- ▼ regular, rapid carotid pulse at 120
- ▼ regular, rapid radial pulse at 120
- ▼ capillary refill at 3 seconds
- ▼ no obvious external blood loss

DISABILITY

- ▼ (A, V, P, U) unresponsive

EXPOSE AND EXAMINE

- ▼ no obvious deformity or discoloration
- ▼ skin turgor fair
- ▼ skin color flushed
- ▼ skin hot and dry to touch
- ▼ weight estimated at 160 lb

SECONDARY ASSESSMENT FINDINGS

VITAL SIGNS

- ▼ respirations, 30 and snoring
- ▼ pulse, 120 and regular

- ▼ blood pressure, 128/78
- ▼ ECG, a sinus tachycardia

HISTORY

- ▼ as above, except for the following:
    - ▼ A unknown
    - ▼ M unknown
    - ▼ P unknown
    - ▼ L unknown
    - ▼ E drinking heavily the night before

HEAD

- ▼ no visible trauma
- ▼ no deformity on palpation
- ▼ pupils equal and reactive
- ▼ no CSF noted
- ▼ no Battle's signs or raccoon's eyes

NECK

- ▼ trachea midline
- ▼ neck veins flat
- ▼ no deformity
- ▼ no discoloration

CHEST

- ▼ no visible deformity
- ▼ no discoloration
- ▼ symmetrical chest wall movement
- ▼ lung sounds clear and equal bilaterally
- ▼ no deformity, tenderness, or crepitus on palpation

ABDOMEN

- ▼ abdomen nondistended
- ▼ soft, nontender to palpation
- ▼ (if checked, bowel sounds present)
- ▼ pelvic rock stable

EXTREMITIES

- ▼ no deformity
- ▼ no discoloration

- ▼ no visible signs of trauma
- ▼ capillary refill at 3 seconds
- ▼ distal pulses present
- ▼ skin turgor fair
- ▼ skin color flushed
- ▼ skin hot and dry to touch
- ▼ no tenderness, crepitus, or swelling
- ▼ no movement of extremities

NEUROLOGICAL

- ▼ unconscious, unresponsive
- ▼ Glascow coma scale calculated at 3:
    - ▼ eye opening, none (1)
    - ▼ verbal response, none (1)
    - ▼ motor response, none (1)

SENSORY EXAM

- ▼ unable to determine motor or sensory function

BACK

- ▼ no deformity
- ▼ no discoloration
- ▼ no trauma noted

Scenario Progression and Analysis: This patient is suffering from heat stroke. EMT-As and Is should be tested on how quickly they diagnose the problem, initiate the airway management, cool the patient, and transport or call for ALS assistance. A twist for the EMTs will be that the patient will later go into cardiac arrest after a seizure. The emphasis for them will be to treat the cardiac arrest within the limits of their local protocols. Paramedics should be tested on how quickly they diagnose the hyperthermia, properly control the airway, hyperventilate, and initiate treatment, including cooling the patient. Midway through the scenario this patient will begin to have a grand mal seizure, which should be treated with diazepam. If the diagnosis and treatment are completed rapidly, the patient's condition will remain the same. If this treatment is not instituted in a timely fashion, the patient should develop status epilepticus and eventually go into cardiac arrest.

SUGGESTED TREATMENT

EMT-A Level

- ▼ Conduct Scene Survey.

- ▾ Remove patient to cooler area.
- ▾ Remove clothes.
▾ Conduct Primary Assessment.
▾ Airway management should include proper application of the bag-valve-mask device with 100% O_2 administration.
  - ▾ Position patient properly.
  - ▾ Open airway with modified jaw thrust method.
  - ▾ Insert naso/oropharyngeal airway.
▾ Cool patient, as per local protocols.
▾ Reassess airway, breathing, circulation, and level of consciousness.

AT THIS TIME, THIS PATIENT HAS A GRAND MAL SEIZURE.

▾ Continue to cool and hyperventilate patient.
  - ▾ Protect patient from injuring himself.

THE SEIZURE STOPS.

▾ Reassess airway, breathing, circulation, and level of consciousness.

THE PATIENT IS NOW APNEIC AND PULSELESS.

▾ Initiate proper CPR.
  - ▾ 5 to 1 ratio of compressions to ventilations.
  - ▾ 80 to 100 compressions per minute.
  - ▾ Proper hand placement and depth of compression.
▾ Consider maintaining cervical spine manually during and after airway management, as per local protocols.
▾ Consider securing patient with cervical immobilization devices to backboard, as per local protocols.
▾ Transport ASAP or call for an ALS Unit.
▾ Conduct Secondary Assessment.
▾ Notify appropriate receiving facility

EMT-I Level

▾ Treatment is the same as above, but includes the following: ⁄
▾ Apply automatic external defibrillator, as per local protocols.
▾ Airway management should include insertion of an esophageal airway.
  - ▾ Place in sniffing position.
  - ▾ Assess lung sounds.
▾ Establish a large-bore IV, infusing normal saline, as per local protocols, KVO.

EMT-P Level

- ▼ Conduct Scene Survey.
- ▼ Conduct Primary Assessment, which includes rapid assessment of ECG, showing a sinus tachycardia.
- ▼ Airway management should include proper application of the bag-valve-mask device with 100% O_2 administration.
    - ▼ Position patient properly.
    - ▼ Open airway with modified jaw thrust method.
    - ▼ Insert naso/oropharyngeal airway.
- ▼ Complete oral intubation with appropriate-sized tube.
    - ▼ Hyperventilate before and after
    - ▼ No longer than 30 seconds
    - ▼ Assess lung sounds.
- ▼ Cool patient, as per local protocols.
- ▼ Reassess airway, breathing, circulation, and level of consciousness.
- ▼ Consider maintaining cervical spine manually during and after airway management, as per local protocols.
- ▼ Conduct Secondary Assessment.
- ▼ Establish a large-bore IV, infusing normal saline, as per local protocols, KVO.
- ▼ Draw blood sample and obtain glucometer/glucostrip reading.

GLUCOSE READING = 68 MG/DL.

- ▼ Administer 50% dextrose, IV.

AT THIS TIME, THE PATIENT HAS A GRAND MAL SEIZURE.

- ▼ Continue to hyperventilate and cool patient.
- ▼ Administer 2.5 to 5 mg of diazepam, as per local protocols.

THE PATIENT STOPS SEIZING.

- ▼ Reassess airway, breathing, circulation, and level of consciousness.
- ▼ Consider securing patient with cervical immobilization devices to backboard, as per local protocols.
- ▼ Administer 2 mg of naloxone, IV.
- ▼ Transport ASAP.
- ▼ Notify appropriate receiving facility.

ADDITIONAL PROBLEMS

Depending on the level of the candidate, the following problems can be added to the scenario:

1. The patient's airway may be made more difficult to manage because of a clenched jaw (that is, nasal intubation, not oral, allowed, and so on).

2. Even though the history is directed toward hyperthermia, the patient could respond to treatment for unknown origin because of narcotics or hypoglycemia.
3. If an oropharyngeal airway is not in place during the seizure, the patient can obstruct the ET tube during the seizure.
4. The patient may vomit prior to airway control.
5. Cooling of the patient may be delayed if proper supplies are not carried. The patient's status should deteriorate if this occurs.
6 Any scene hazard can be incorporated, at the presenter's discretion. (This is in addition to or replacement of those already mentioned.)
7. Even after the proper treatment has been accomplished, the patient can still deteriorate and go into cardiac arrest to further test the candidate's knowledge.
8. When diazepam is administered, the patient can go into respiratory arrest.
9. The presenter may add any underlying medical problems that he or she wishes to test (for example heart disease or hypertension).
10. Any location can be given to test the candidate's street or address competency, using local running cards.
11. If universal precautions are not followed, the candidate can be told, after the scenario, that the patient had HIV or hepatitis.

SUMMARY

This patient presents with the common symptoms of heat stroke. Heat stroke is a failure of heat regulation controlled centrally by the hypothalmus and not a problem of fluid and electrolyte loss as seen in heat exhaustion. This individual has been in the hot sun with a high humidity, but now appears unconscious with hot and dry skin. The classic presentation of heat stroke is a patient without the normal compensatory mechanism of heat dissipation. Heat loss through evaporation can become ineffective if the patient is in a hot, humid environment. Humidity of greater than 75% significantly reduces heat loss through sweating. This causes a rise in core temperature. As the body's core temperature begins to rise, the metabolism and subsequent heat production begins to increase, as well. Soon the patient suffers from heat stroke. Drugs, including alcohol, can suppress the hypothalmus. If this occurs, thermoregulatory failure will follow, especially if the patient is in this kind of environment.

The patient may present with the above physical findings. Additionally, seizures can occur in the presence of increased body temperature. Treatment is begun by removing the patient from the hot environment. The air-conditioned treatment area of a rescue vehicle is ideal to begin the cooling process. Application of ice to the groin, head, and axilla will also help. Cooling of IV fluids may aid in reducing central body temperature.

Because the patient has a history of previous alcohol ingestion, hypoglycemia should be considered. If the tests for hypoglycemia confirm low glucose, correct treatment should be initiated.

MEDICAL SCENARIO 7

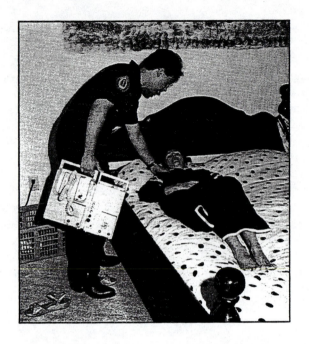

Type: medical—dehydration.
Scenario moulage/prop list: Live model or mannequin, bed, talc for poor skin turgor, grease paint for pale skin color (bedroom setting).

INITIAL SCENE DESCRIPTION

Dispatch Information

LOCATION: Apartment in a congregate living facility
NUMBER OF VICTIMS: 1
TYPE OF SITUATION: Nausea and vomiting
HAZARDS: NONE
WEATHER CONDITIONS: Warm, sunny afternoon
TIME OF DAY: 1425 hours

Scene

You arrive on scene at the apartment of a 68-year-old woman in a congregate living facility. Her door is open and, after announcing yourself, she tells you to enter. You find the woman lying supine on her bed. She states, "I have been nauseous for 3 days and can't keep anything down." She goes on to explain that she is now very weak and dizzy upon standing. You inquire about blood in the vomitus and she answers that it appeared to be normal.

PRIMARY ASSESSMENT FINDINGS

SCENE SURVEY

▼ apartment with woman lying in bed
▼ no apparent hazards

AIRWAY/CERVICAL SPINE

▼ airway open
▼ no signs of trauma
▼ neck veins flat

BREATHING

▼ 28 breaths per minute
▼ symmetrical chest rise
▼ lung sounds clear bilaterally

CIRCULATION/HEMORRHAGE CONTROL

▼ regular, carotid pulse at 64
▼ regular, radial pulse at 64
▼ capillary refill delayed to 4 seconds
▼ no obvious external blood loss

DISABILITY

▼ (A, V, P, U) alert

EXPOSE AND EXAMINE

▼ no obvious deformity or discoloration
▼ skin turgor poor
▼ skin color pale
▼ skin cool and dry to touch
▼ weight estimated at 150 lb

SECONDARY ASSESSMENT FINDINGS

VITAL SIGNS

▼ respirations, 28
▼ pulse, 64 and regular
▼ blood pressure, 78/50
▼ ECG, a normal sinus rhythm

HISTORY

▼ as above, except for the following:

- ▼ A penicillin
- ▼ M propranolol and furosemide
- ▼ P hypertension, glaucoma
- ▼ L 3 days ago
- ▼ E nausea and vomiting

HEAD

- ▼ no visible trauma
- ▼ no deformity on palpation
- ▼ right pupil midpoint and reactive
- ▼ left pupil irregular and nonreactive due to surgery

NECK

- ▼ trachea midline
- ▼ neck veins flat
- ▼ no deformity
- ▼ no discoloration

CHEST

- ▼ no visible deformity
- ▼ no discoloration
- ▼ symmetrical chest wall movement
- ▼ lung sounds clear and equal bilaterally
- ▼ no deformity, tenderness, or crepitus on palpation

ABDOMEN

- ▼ abdomen nondistended
- ▼ soft, nontender to palpation
- ▼ no masses palpated
- ▼ (if checked, bowel sounds present)
- ▼ pelvic rock stable

EXTREMITIES

- ▼ no deformity
- ▼ no discoloration
- ▼ no visible signs of trauma
- ▼ capillary refill 4 seconds
- ▼ distal pulses present
- ▼ skin turgor poor
- ▼ skin pale
- ▼ skin cool and dry to touch
- ▼ no tenderness, crepitus, or swelling
- ▼ movement of extremities equal

NEUROLOGICAL

- ▾ conscious, alert
- ▾ Glasgow coma scale calculated at 15:
    - ▾ eye opening, spontaneous (4)
    - ▾ verbal response, oriented (5)
    - ▾ motor response, obeys (6)

SENSORY EXAM

- ▾ no deficit in sensory or motor function

BACK

- ▾ no deformity
- ▾ no discoloration
- ▾ no trauma noted

Scenario Progression and Analysis: This patient is suffering from dehydration after experiencing episodes of nausea and vomiting for 3 days. Despite a normal pulse rate, this patient is severely hypovolemic. Her hypertensive medication prevents an increase in heart rate that would normally compensate for decreased volume. EMT-As should be tested on how quickly they diagnose the problem, initiate airway management for the patient, apply the pneumatic antishock trousers, and transport or call for ALS assistance. The EMT-Is, like the paramedics, should be tested on how quickly they diagnose the problem, properly control the airway, and initiate treatment, including volume and electrolyte replacement. If both the diagnosis and treatment are completed rapidly, the patient's condition will improve; if not, her condition should deteriorate.

SUGGESTED TREATMENT

EMT-A Level

- ▾ Conduct Scene Survey.
- ▾ Conduct Primary Assessment.
- ▾ Airway management should include high-flow O_2 administration with a mask.
- ▾ Place patient in Trendelenburg.
- ▾ Reassess airway, breathing, circulation, and level of consciousness.

PATIENT'S BP = 78/50.

- ▾ Conduct MAST survey and then apply pneumatic antishock trousers as per protocols.
- ▾ Reassess airway, breathing, circulation, and level of consciousness.

PATIENT'S BP = 100/60.

- Transport or call for an ALS Unit.
- Conduct Secondary Assessment.
- Notify appropriate receiving facility.

EMT-I Level

- Treatment is the same as above (except for the application of the pneumatic antishock garment) and includes the following:
- Establish a large–bore IV, infusing Ringer's normal saline or lactate, open.
    - 200 cc fluid bolus.
- Reassess airway, breathing, circulation, and level of consciousness.

PATIENT'S BP = 86/58.

- Repeat fluid bolus of 200 cc.
- Reassess airway, breathing, circulation, and level of consciousness.

PATIENT'S BP = 96/64.

EMT-P Level

- Conduct Scene Survey.
- Conduct Primary Assessment.
- Airway management should include high-flow O_2 administration with a mask.
- Assess ECG, showing a normal sinus rhythm.
- Conduct Secondary Assessment.
- Establish one large-bore IV infusing Ringer's normal saline or lactate, open.
    - 200 cc fluid bolus.
- Reassess airway, breathing, circulation, and level of consciousness.
- Draw blood sample and obtain glucometer/glucostrip reading since patient has been vomiting for three days.

GLUCOSE READING = 80 MG/DL.
PATIENT'S BP = 86/58.

- Repeat fluid bolus of 200 cc.
- Reassess airway, breathing, circulation, and level of consciousness.

PATIENT'S BP = 96/64.

- Transport.
- Notify appropriate receiving facility.

ADDITIONAL PROBLEMS

Depending on the level of the candidate, the following problems can be added to the scenario:

1. The patient may experience cardiac dysrhythmias due to hypokalemia.
2. Even though the history is directed toward dehydration, the patient could respond to treatment for hypoglycemia.
3. The patient may again vomit with aspiration and subsequent respiratory arrest.
4. Any scene hazard can be incorporated at the presenter's discretion. (This is in addition to or replacement of those already mentioned.)
5. Even after the proper treatment has been accomplished, the patient can still deteriorate and go into cardiac arrest to further test the candidate's knowledge.
6. Additional boluses, or even pneumatic antishock garment application, can be required before the patient's blood pressure increases significantly.
7. The presenter may include other additional, underlying medical problems that he or she wishes to test (for example, epilepsy or COPD).
8. Any location can be given to test the candidate's street or address competency, using local running cards.

SUMMARY

This patient has been vomiting for several days, making her unable to replace lost fluids. This condition has been further complicated by her already tenuous volume and electrolyte status from furosemide use. The volume and electrolyte imbalance can cause cardiac dysrhythmias for any patient in this situation. The main direction of treatment should be aimed toward replacement of lost fluid volume and electrolytes. Any volume replacement requires careful observation for pulmonary edema in the elderly patient. The patient's airway should be carefully observed because of possible continued vomiting and the potential for aspiration.

Because she was on the beta blocker propranolol, her pulse remained constant at 64 instead of increasing as it would normally do to compensate for the fluid loss.

Chapter 3

OBSTETRICAL SCENARIOS

OBSTETRICAL SCENARIO 1

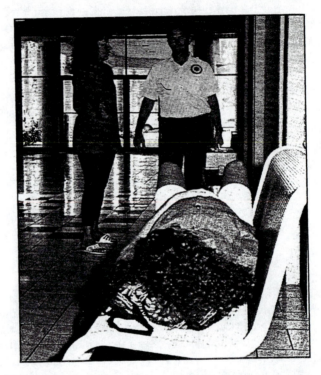

Type: Obstetric.
Scenario moulage/prop list: Live model or mannequin, live model
for mother's role, pillow, simulated blood, grease paint for pale skin
color, glycerin water for skin (mall setting).

INITIAL SCENE DESCRIPTION

Dispatch Information

LOCATION: The mall
NUMBER OF VICTIMS: 1
TYPE OF SITUATION: Bleeding
HAZARDS: None
WEATHER CONDITIONS: Clear evening
TIME OF DAY: 2000 hours

Scene

You are en route to this call of "bleeding" when the dispatch calls you back, informing you that this patient is a 20-year-old female who is eight months pregnant. A frantic woman meets you out in front of the mall just as you step down from your truck. She says that her daughter is having severe abdominal pain with some vaginal bleeding.

You arrive at a bench within the mall and find the 20- year-old patient lying supine on the bench and breathing rapidly, with a weak, rapid carotid pulse. She appears alert and says she is under no prenatal care.

PRIMARY ASSESSMENT FINDINGS

SCENE SURVEY

▼ woman lying on bench in a public mall
▼ a frantic mother

AIRWAY/CERVICAL SPINE

▼ airway open
▼ no signs of trauma
▼ neck veins flat

BREATHING

▼ 32 breaths per minute
▼ symmetrical chest rise
▼ lung sounds clear bilaterally

CIRCULATION/HEMORRHAGE CONTROL

▼ regular, carotid pulse at 136
▼ no radial pulse
▼ capillary refill delayed to 4 seconds
▼ scant external blood loss from vagina

DISABILITY

▼ (A, V, P, U) alert, but becoming sluggish

EXPOSE AND EXAMINE

▼ obviously pregnant
▼ skin turgor good
▼ skin color pale
▼ skin cool and diaphoretic to touch
▼ weight estimated at 142 lb.

SECONDARY ASSESSMENT FINDINGS

VITAL SIGNS

- respirations , 32
- pulse, 136 and regular
- blood pressure, 78/50
- ECG, a sinus tachycardia without ectopy

HISTORY

- as above, except for the following:
    - A   none
    - M   none
    - P   8 months pregnant, gravida 4, para 1
    - L   normal dinner that evening, 1 hour ago
    - E   walking around mall

HEAD

- no visible trauma
- no deformity on palpation
- pupils equal and reactive to light

NECK

- trachea midline
- neck veins flat
- no deformity
- no discoloration

CHEST

- no visible deformity
- no discoloration
- symmetrical chest wall movement
- lung sounds clear and equal bilaterally
- breast enlargement and tenderness noted

ABDOMEN

- fundus is noted midway between umbilicus and xiphoid process
- abdomen distended with no contractions noted
- rigid and extremely tender to palpation
- fetal heart tones present at a rate of 90
- external vaginal exam reveals minimal bleeding
- no crowning noted

EXTREMITIES

- ▼ no deformity
- ▼ no discoloration
- ▼ no visible signs of trauma
- ▼ capillary refill delayed to 4 seconds
- ▼ no distal pulses present
- ▼ skin turgor good
- ▼ skin cool and diaphoretic to touch
- ▼ no tenderness, crepitus, or swelling
- ▼ sluggish but equal movement of extremities

NEUROLOGICAL

- ▼ conscious, alert, but becoming progressively more sluggish
- ▼ Glascow coma scale calculated at 15:
    - ▼ eye opening, spontaneous (4)
    - ▼ verbal response, oriented (5)
    - ▼ motor response, obeys (6)

SENSORY EXAM

- ▼ sluggish, but no deficit in sensory or motor function

BACK

- ▼ no deformity
- ▼ no discoloration
- ▼ no trauma noted

Scenario Progression and Analysis: This patient is in hypovolemic shock due to third trimester bleeding. All EMTs should be tested on how quickly they diagnose the problem, properly control the airway, administer oxygen, apply the pneumatic antishock garment (excluding the abdominal section), and transport or call for an ALS Unit. IV administration should also be looked at for the EMT-Is and paramedics. If rapidly diagnosed and properly treated, this patient's condition will remain the same; if not, her condition should deteriorate.

UGGESTED TREATMENT

EMT-A Level

- ▼ Conduct Scene Survey.
    - ▼ Remove or calm patient's mother.
- ▼ Conduct Primary Assessment.
- ▼ Recognize this as a true obstetrical emergency and transport rapidly or call for an ALS Unit.

- Airway management should include high-flow O_2 administration with a mask.
- Place patient in left lateral recumbent position.
- Reassess airway, breathing, circulation, and level of consciousness.
- Conduct MAST survey and apply the pneumatic anti-shock garment, inflating the legs only as per local protocols.
- Reassess airway, breathing, circulation, and level of consciousness.
- Notify appropriate receiving facility.
- Conduct Secondary Assessment.

EMT-I Level

- Treatment is the same as above, but includes the following:
- Establish at least two large-bore IVs infusing Ringer's lactate, open.
- Reassess airway, breathing, circulation, and level of consciousness.

EMT-P Level

- Conduct Scene Survey.
  - Remove or calm patient's mother.
- Conduct Primary Assessment.
- Airway management should include high-flow O_2 administration with a mask.
- Place patient in left lateral recumbent position.
- Reassess airway, breathing, circulation, and level of consciousness.
- Conduct MAST Survey and apply the pneumatic anti-shock garment, inflating the legs only as per local protocols.
- Reassess airway, breathing, circulation, and level of consciousness.
- Transport ASAP.
- Establish at least two large bore IVs infusing Ringer's lactate, open.
- Reassess airway, breathing, circulation, and level of consciousness.
- Conduct Secondary Assessment.
- Notify appropriate receiving facility.

ADDITIONAL PROBLEMS

Depending on the level of the candidate, the following problems can be added to the scenario:

1. The patient's blood pressure could deteriorate due to occult hemorrhage even though proper treatment is completed, and cardiac arrest could follow.

2. The patient could deliver a stillborn.

3. The patient could deliver an infant in distress (for example, with meconium aspiration) and significant postpartum hemorrhage could follow.

4. Any scene hazard can be incorporated at the presenter's discretion. (This is in addition to or replacement of those already mentioned.).

5. Additional difficulty of airway management can be accomplished by adding vomiting to the scenario or by requiring the patient to have to be intubated.

6. If the abdominal section of the antishock garment is inflated, the mother should go into respiratory arrest due to abdominal content incursion on the diaphragm.

7. Any location can be given to test the candidate's street or address competency, using local running cards.

8. If this patient is placed in a flat position on the stretcher or backboard, she should become extremely hypotensive and rapidly lose consciousness.

SUMMARY

This patient is suffering from abruptio placentae. Because of the premature separation of the placenta from the uterine wall, massive concealed hemorrhage can occur. This concealed hemorrhage distends the uterus and causes the rigidity and exquisite abdominal tenderness. The location of the separation on the uterine wall and placenta, as well as the location of the fetus in the birth canal, determines the amount of external bleeding. Even though this bleeding may appear slight, the hemorrhage is profound and will lead to maternal shock and eventually death unless the appropriate intervention is rapid. *Remember, the leading cause of fetal death is maternal death.* The candidate must recognize this pathophysiology and minimally prepare the patient for transport to an appropriate facility, that handles obstetrical emergencies of this type. No definitive treatment is available in the prehospital environment and the only definitive treatment is a cesarean section. The survival of both the mother and the unborn child depends greatly on early recognition and rapid transport by the prehospital provider.

OBSTETRICAL SCENARIO 2

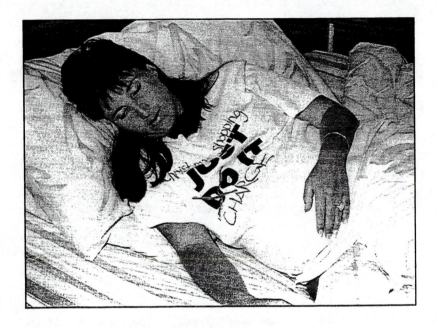

Type: combination—obstetric, pediatric.
Scenario moulage/prop list: Live model or mannequin, pillow, OB delivery mannequin or infant mannequin, glycerin water in spray bottle for skin (living-room setting).

INITIAL SCENE DESCRIPTION

Dispatch Information

LOCATION: Residential house
NUMBER OF VICTIMS: 1
TYPE OF SITUATION: Woman in labor
HAZARDS: None
WEATHER CONDITIONS: Cool, clear evening
TIME OF DAY: 2035 hours

Scene

You are called to the scene of a woman in labor. A friend is on scene and states that the patient, an 18-year-old female, was in active labor when she had a seizure. When you reach the patient, she is extremely lethargic and confused. You note that she has edema in her feet, hands, and around her eyes.

PRIMARY ASSESSMENT FINDINGS

SCENE SURVEY

- ▼ living room in residential home
- ▼ woman lying supine on couch
- ▼ no apparent hazards

AIRWAY/CERVICAL SPINE

- ▼ airway open
- ▼ no signs of trauma
- ▼ necks veins slightly distended

BREATHING

- ▼ 24 breaths per minute
- ▼ symmetrical chest wall movement
- ▼ lung sounds clear bilaterally

CIRCULATION/HEMORRHAGE CONTROL

- ▼ regular, carotid pulse at 100
- ▼ regular, radial pulse at 100
- ▼ capillary refill at 2 seconds
- ▼ scant external blood loss from vagina

DISABILITY

- ▼ (A, V, P, U) responsive to verbal stimuli

EXPOSE AND EXAMINE

- ▼ obviously pregnant
- ▼ skin turgor good
- ▼ skin color normal
- ▼ skin warm and diaphoretic to touch
- ▼ weight estimated at 170 lb

SECONDARY ASSESSMENT FINDINGS

VITAL SIGNS

- ▼ respirations, 24
- ▼ pulse, 100 and regular
- ▼ blood pressure, 150/110
- ▼ ECG, a normal sinus rhythm

HISTORY

▼ as above, except for the following:
  - ▼ A   none
  - ▼ M   no prenatal care
  - ▼ P   full-term pregnancy, first pregnancy, rapid weight gain, preexisting hypertension
  - ▼ L   light breakfast this A.M.
  - ▼ E   in active labor, seizure

HEAD

▼ no visible trauma

▼ edema noted around eyes

▼ no deformity on palpation

▼ pupils equal and reactive to light

NECK

▼ trachea midline

▼ neck veins slightly distended

▼ no deformity

▼ no discoloration

CHEST

▼ no visible deformity

▼ no discoloration

▼ symmetrical chest wall movement

▼ lung sounds clear and equal bilaterally

▼ no crepitus on palpation

▼ breast enlargement and tenderness noted

ABDOMEN

▼ fundus is noted at the level of the xiphoid process

▼ abdomen distended with contractions noted

▼ fetal heart tones present at a rate of 140

▼ baby's buttocks presenting

EXTREMITIES

▼ severe pedal and finger edema noted

▼ no discoloration

▼ no visible signs of trauma

▼ capillary refill at 2 seconds

- distal pulses present
- skin turgor good
- skin warm and diaphoretic to touch
- no tenderness or crepitus
- sluggish but equal movement of extremities

NEUROLOGICAL

- conscious, confused, but becoming progressively more sluggish
- Glascow coma scale calculated at 14:
    - eye opening, spontaneous (4)
    - verbal response, confused (4)
    - motor response, obeys (6)

SENSORY EXAM

- sluggish, but normal sensory and motor function

BACK

- sacral edema noted
- no discoloration
- no trauma noted

Scenario Progression and Analysis: This patient is both eclamptic and about to give birth. She will have another seizure and, later, begin a breech delivery. All EMTs should insert a gloved hand into the patient's vagina once 3 minutes has elapsed and the baby still has not been delivered. EMT-As and Is should be tested on their rapid diagnosis of the problems, support of the mother, proper airway control, and the decision to transport or call for an ALS Unit. Paramedics should administer diazepam for the seizure and rapidly transport, because the baby has not been delivered. If these interventions are completed, the patient will survive. If not, the baby's condition should deteriorate.

SUGGESTED TREATMENT

EMT-A Level

- Conduct Scene Survey.
- Conduct Primary Assessment.
- Airway management should include high-flow O_2 administration with a mask.
- Place patient in proper position for delivery.
- Conduct Secondary Assessment.

AT THIS TIME, THE PATIENT HAS A GRAND MAL SEIZURE.

- Protect patient.
  - Loosen clothes.
- Airway management should include proper application of the bag-valve-mask device with 100% O_2 administration.
  - Position patient properly.
  - Open airway with head-tilt, chin-lift.
  - Insert naso/oropharyngeal airway.

THE SEIZURE STOPS AND PATIENT REMAINS UNCONSCIOUS.

- Reassess airway, breathing, circulation, and level of consciousness.

AT THIS TIME, THE PATIENT'S CONTRACTIONS CONTINUE, BUT ONLY THE LEGS AND BUTTOCKS OF THE BABY PRESENT.

- Support baby's buttocks and extremities.
- Recognize this as a true obstetrical emergency and transport rapidly or call for an ALS Unit.
- Reassess airway, breathing, circulation, and level of consciousness (of mother).

THREE MINUTES ELAPSE AND STILL THE BABY HAS NOT BEEN DELIVERED.

- Insert a gloved hand and form a V around the infant's nose.
- Notify appropriate receiving facility.

EMT-I Level

- Treatment is the same as above, but includes the following:
- Airway management should include insertion of an esophageal airway, since the patient remains unconscious.
  - Place in sniffing position.
  - Assess lung sounds.
- Establish a large-bore IV of Ringer's lactate, as per local protocols, KVO.

EMT-P Level

- Conduct Scene Survey.
- Conduct Primary Assessment.

- Airway management should include high-flow O_2 administration with a mask.
- Place patient in proper position for delivery.
- Establish a large-bore IV of Ringer's lactate, as per local protocols, KVO.
- Conduct Secondary Assessment.

AT THIS TIME, THE PATIENT HAS
A GRAND MAL SEIZURE.

- Protect patient.
  - Loosen clothes.
- Airway management should include proper application of the bag-valve-mask device with 100% O_2 administration.
  - Position patient properly.
  - Open airway with head-tilt, chin-lift.
  - Insert naso/oropharyngeal airway.
- Administer 2.5 + 5 mg of diazepam or as per local protocols.
- Administer 1G of 20% solution of magnesium sulfate, over 5 minutes IV, if carried, to prevent further seizures or as per local protocols.

THE SEIZURE STOPS AND PATIENT REMAINS
UNCONSCIOUS.

- Reassess airway, breathing, circulation, and level of consciousness.
- Complete oral intubation with appropriate-sized tube.
  - Hyperventilate before and after.
  - No longer than 30 seconds.
  - Assess lung sounds.

AT THIS TIME, THE PATIENT'S CONTRACTIONS
CONTINUE, BUT ONLY THE LEGS AND BUTTOCKS
OF THE BABY PRESENT.

- Support baby's buttocks and extremities.
- Transport ASAP.
- Reassess airway, breathing, circulation, and level of consciousness (of mother).

THREE MINUTES ELAPSE AND STILL THE BABY
HAS NOT BEEN DELIVERED.

- Insert a gloved hand and form a V around the infant's nose.
- Notify appropriate receiving facility.

ADDITIONAL PROBLEMS

Depending on the level of the candidate, the following problems can be added to the scenario:

1. The patient's blood pressure could deteriorate due to occult hemorrhage.
2. The patient could eventually deliver an infant in distress (for example, from meconium aspiration) and significant postpartum hemorrhage could follow.
3. The patient could have another seizure, requiring more diazepam.
4. The patient could go into respiratory arrest or depression because of the administration of the diazepam.
5. This baby could deliver and be the first of twins.
6. Any scene hazard can be incorporated at the presenter's discretion. (This is in addition to or replacement of those already mentioned.)
7. Additional difficulty of airway management can be accomplished by adding vomiting to the scenario.
8. Even though the correct treatment is accomplished, the patient may still seize and deteriorate into cardiac arrest.
9. The presenter may add any other additional medical problems that he or she wishes to test (for example, hypoglycemia or epilepsy).
10. Any location can be given to test the candidate's street or address competency, using local running cards.

SUMMARY

This scenario presents the candidate with multiple problems associated with the obstetrical patient. The patient suffers from eclampsia. The exact pathophysiology of this disease is unknown. The only known cure is delivery of the fetus. This condition occurs in the obstetrical patient in the third trimester in 5% to 6% of all pregnancies. It is usually associated with the first pregnancy and is commonly seen in those females who are younger than 18 or older than 35 years of age. Some predisposing factors that can contribute to the development of eclampsia are preexisting hypertension, diabetes, dietary deficiencies, and, a family history of this pathology. The diagnosis of preeclampsia is made when the sustained BP is greater than 140/90. The signs and symptoms seen with preeclampsia include tachycardia, petechiae, and facial, hand, and pedal edema, as well as visual disturbances. The patient may complain that her jewelry or shoes "don't fit anymore" or "are too tight." This should alert the prehospital provider to the possibility of preeclampsia. Eclampsia is all of the above signs and symptoms with the addition of seizure activity and possibly coma. Only about 5% of the preeclampsia cases progress to the eclamptic state. Once the patient is eclamptic, she has a 2% to 5% chance of maternal mortality and her baby, a 10% to 37% chance of fetal mortality. Some complications include disseminated intravascular coagulation, cerebral hemorrhage, abruptio placentae, pulmonary edema and hepatic necrosis. Treatment for these is directed toward reducing seizure activity and preventing maternal and fetal hypoxia.

Magnesium sulfate, although rarely carried now in the prehospital setting, is effective in controlling and preventing seizure activity in the eclamptic patient, and it may be more widely used in the future for certain cardiac dysrhythmias.

In addition to the eclampsia, the mother presents with a breech delivery that will not deliver. This emergency cannot be managed in the prehospital setting and requires a cesarean section. Early recognition and rapid transport are required to reduce the potential of fetal and/or maternal mortality.

OBSTETRICAL SCENARIO 3

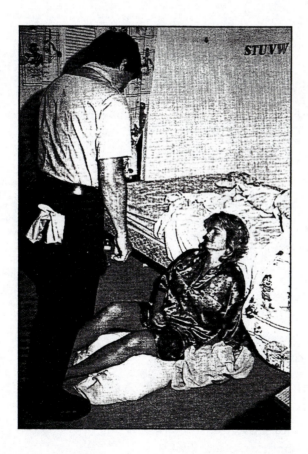

Type: Combination—obstetric, pediatric.
Scenario moulage/prop list: Live model or mannequin for mother's role, infant mannequin, grease paint for pale skin color, simulated blood, glycerin water for skin (one-room apartment setting).

INITIAL SCENE DESCRIPTION

Dispatch Information

LOCATION: Apartment in the city
NUMBER OF VICTIMS: Possibly 2
TYPE OF SITUATION: Woman who has just had a baby
HAZARDS: None
WEATHER CONDITIONS: Cool, snowy afternoon
TIME OF DAY: 1600 hours

Scene

You are dispatched to an apartment in the city for a problem involving two patients, a mother and her newborn. En route, you attempt to have another unit respond, but you're the only rescue truck available. Upon arrival, the person who called 911, the apartment manager, directs you to the patients. There you find the mother sitting on the floor with the newborn, who is wrapped in a towel beside her, not moving. The umbilical cord still joins them. The mother is somewhat sluggish, but crying. There is a moderate amount of blood loss in the area.

PRIMARY ASSESSMENT FINDINGS:
PATIENT 1, THE MOTHER

SCENE SURVEY

- residential home
- woman sitting up
- no apparent hazards

AIRWAY/CERVICAL SPINE

- airway open
- no signs of trauma
- neck veins flat

BREATHING

- 24 breaths per minute
- symmetrical chest rise
- lung sounds clear bilaterally

CIRCULATION/HEMORRHAGE CONTROL

- regular, carotid pulse at 132
- no radial pulse

- ▼ capillary refill delayed to 5 seconds
- ▼ moderate external blood loss from vagina

DISABILITY

- ▼ (A, V, P, U) responsive to verbal stimuli

EXPOSE AND EXAMINE

- ▼ no obvious deformity or discoloration
- ▼ skin turgor good
- ▼ skin color pale
- ▼ skin cool and diaphoretic to touch
- ▼ weight estimated at 145 lb

SECONDARY ASSESSMENT FINDINGS: PATIENT 1, THE MOTHER

VITAL SIGNS

- ▼ respirations, 24 and shallow
- ▼ pulse, 132 and regular
- ▼ blood pressure, 70/40
- ▼ ECG, a sinus tachycardia rhythm

HISTORY

- ▼ as above, except for the following:
  - ▼ A unknown
  - ▼ M unknown
  - ▼ P unknown
  - ▼ L unknown
  - ▼ E in active labor with birth prior to your arrival

HEAD

- ▼ no visible trauma
- ▼ no deformity on palpation
- ▼ pupils equal and reactive to light

NECK

- ▼ trachea midline
- ▼ neck veins flat
- ▼ no deformity
- ▼ no discoloration

CHEST

- ▾ no visible deformity
- ▾ no discoloration
- ▾ symmetrical chest wall movement
- ▾ lung sounds are clear and equal bilaterally
- ▾ no crepitus on palpation
- ▾ breast enlargement and tenderness noted

ABDOMEN

- ▾ flat, no visual deformity
- ▾ nontender, boggy to palpation
- ▾ external vaginal exam reveals moderate bleeding and umbilical cord
- ▾ no crowning noted, at this time

EXTREMITIES

- ▾ no deformity noted
- ▾ no discoloration
- ▾ no visible signs of trauma
- ▾ capillary refill delayed to 5 seconds
- ▾ no distal pulses present
- ▾ skin turgor good
- ▾ skin color pale
- ▾ skin cool and diaphoretic to touch
- ▾ no tenderness or crepitus
- ▾ movement of extremities equal

NEUROLOGICAL

- ▾ conscious, but becoming progressively more sluggish
- ▾ Glascow coma scale calculated at 14:
    - ▾ eye opening, spontaneous (4)
    - ▾ verbal response, confused (4)
    - ▾ motor response, obeys (6)

SENSORY EXAM

- ▾ no deficit in sensory or motor function

BACK

- ▾ no deformity noted
- ▾ no discoloration
- ▾ no trauma noted

Scenario Progression and Analysis: This patient is suffering from hypovolemic shock after delivering a baby. All EMTs should cut the cord and have the mother massage her fundus. EMT-As and Is should be tested on their rapid diagnosis of the problems, support of the mother with proper airway control, application of the pneumatic antishock garment and the decision to transport or call for an ALS Unit. EMT-Is and paramedics should initiate at least two large-bore IVs, as well. If rapidly diagnosed and properly treated, this patient should remain the same. If not, her condition should deteriorate.

PRIMARY ASSESSMENT FINDINGS:
PATIENT 2, THE BABY

SCENE SURVEY

▼ residential home
▼ wrapped in towel
▼ no apparent hazards

AIRWAY/CERVICAL SPINE

▼ airway open
▼ neck veins flat

BREATHING

▼ 30 breaths per minute
▼ symmetrical chest rise
▼ lung sounds reveal rhonchi bilaterally

CIRCULATION/HEMORRHAGE CONTROL

▼ regular, brachial pulse at 60
▼ capillary refill delayed to 4 seconds
▼ no external blood loss

DISABILITY

▼ (A, V, P, U) responsive only to painful stimuli

EXPOSE AND EXAMINE

▼ apparently just delivered
▼ skin turgor good
▼ skin color pale with cyanotic extremities
▼ skin cool and moist to touch (amniotic fluid)
▼ weight estimated at 7 lb

SECONDARY ASSESSMENT FINDINGS:
PATIENT 2, THE BABY

VITAL SIGNS

- respirations, 30 and shallow
- pulse, 60 and regular
- blood pressure, unable to obtain
- ECG, a sinus rhythm

HISTORY

- as above except for the following
  - A   unknown
  - M   none
  - P   none
  - L   none
  - E   delivered prior to your arrival

HEAD

- no visible trauma
- no deformity on palpation
- cyanosis around lips
- meconium noted around mouth
- pupils equal and reactive to light

NECK

- trachea midline
- neck veins flat
- no deformity
- no discoloration

CHEST

- no visible deformity
- no discoloration
- symmetrical chest wall movement
- lung sounds reveal rhonchi bilaterally

ABDOMEN

- no visible deformity
- nontender to palpation
- attached cord

EXTREMITIES

- no deformity noted
- cyanosis noted to arms and legs
- no visible signs of trauma
- capillary refill delayed to 4 seconds
- no distal pulses present
- skin turgor good
- color pale and cyanotic
- skin cool and dry to touch
- no tenderness or crepitus
- no movement of extremities noted

NEUROLOGICAL

- unconscious
- APGAR score is 4:
    - activity, limp (0)
    - pulse, 100 (1)
    - grimace, some flexion (1)
    - appearance, blue/pale (1)
    - respirations, slow(1)

SENSORY EXAM

- some sensory and motor function

BACK

- no deformity noted
- no discoloration
- no trauma noted

Scenario Progression and Analysis: This infant is stressed because the delivery involved meconium aspiration. CPR should be started immediately on this patient, along with vigorous and thorough suctioning. The patient should also be stimulated and warmed. If PALS guidelines are followed, the infant should improve.

SUGGESTED TREATMENT FOR PATIENT 1, THE MOTHER

EMT-A Level

- Conduct Scene Survey.
- Conduct Primary Assessment.

- Airway management should include high-flow O_2 administration with a mask.
- Place patient in Trendelenburg and initiate a fundal massage.
- Reassess airway, breathing, circulation, and level of consciousness.
- Conduct MAST Survey and apply the pneumatic antishock garment, all fields as per local protocols.
- Reassess airway, breathing, circulation, and level of consciousness.
- Transport ASAP or call for an ALS Unit.
- Conduct Secondary Asessment and cut and clamp umbilical cord.
- Notify appropriate facility.

EMT-I Level

- Treatment is the same as above, but includes the following:
- Establish at least two large-bore IVs infusing Ringer's lactate, open.
- Reassess airway, breathing, circulation, and level of consciousness.

EMT-P Level:

- Conduct Scene Survey.
- Conduct Primary Assessment.
- Airway management should include high-flow O_2 administration with a mask.
- Place patient in Trendelenburg and initiate a fundal massage.
- Reassess airway, breathing, circulation, and level of consciousness.
- Conduct MAST Survey and apply the pneumatic anti-shock garment, all fields as per local protocols.
- Reassess airway, breathing, circulation and level of consciousness.
- Transport ASAP.
- Conduct Secondary Assessment and cut and clamp umbilical cord.
- Establish at least two large-bore IVs infusing Ringer's lactate, open.
- Notify appropriate receiving facility.

SUGGESTED TREATMENT FOR PATIENT 2, THE BABY

EMT-A Level

- Conduct Scene Survey.
- Conduct Primary Assessment.
- Suction vigorously.
  - Hyperventilate before and after.
  - Suction orally and nasally with bulb syringe.

▼ Airway management should include proper application of the bag-valve-mask device with 100% O_2 administration.
   ▼ Position patient properly.
   ▼ Open airway with head-tilt, chin-lift.
   ▼ Insert oropharyngeal airway.
▼ Assure that patient is wrapped warmly.
▼ Stimulate and position patient.
▼ Reassess airway, breathing, circulation, and level of consciousness.
▼ Initiate proper CPR.
   ▼ Two finger compressions, one fingerbreadth below the nipple line.
   ▼ At least 100 compressions per minute.
   ▼ Proper depth of compression.
▼ Transport ASAP or call for an ALS Unit.
▼ Reassess airway, breathing, circulation, and level of consciousness.

AT THIS TIME THE INFANT'S COLOR IS PINKER AND HIS PULSE RATE IS 100.

▼ Discontinue CPR and conduct Secondary Assessment.
▼ Clamp and cut umbilical cord.
▼ Notify appropriate facility.

EMT-I Level

▼ Treatment is the same as above, but includes the following:
▼ Establish an IV of dextrose 10%, as per local protocols, KVO.

EMT-P Level

▼ Conduct Scene Survey.
▼ Conduct Primary Assessment.
▼ Suction vigorously.
   ▼ Hyperventilate before and after.
   ▼ Suction orally and nasally with bulb syringe.
   ▼ Deep tracheal suctioning should be performed, initially with ET tube.
▼ Airway management should include proper application of the bag-valve-mask device with 100% O_2 administration.
   ▼ Position patient properly.
   ▼ Open airway with head-tilt, chin-lift.
   ▼ Insert oropharyngeal airway.
▼ Assure that patient is wrapped warmly.
▼ Stimulate and position patient.
▼ Reassess airway, breathing, circulation, and level of consciousness.

- ▼ Initiate proper CPR.
  - ▼ Two finger compressions, one fingerbreadth below the nipple line.
  - ▼ At least 100 compressions per minute.
  - ▼ proper depth of compression.
- ▼ Transport ASAP.
- ▼ Reassess airway, breathing, circulation, and level of consciousness.

**AT THIS TIME THE INFANT'S COLOR IS PINKER
AND HIS PULSE RATE IS 100.**

- ▼ Discontinue CPR and conduct Secondary Assessment.
- ▼ Notify appropriate facility.
- ▼ Clamp and cut umbilical cord.
- ▼ Establish an IV of dextrose 10%, as per local protocols, KVO.

ADDITIONAL PROBLEMS

Depending on the level of the candidate, the following problems can be added to the scenario:

1. Because of continued postpartum hemorrhage, the mother can become more hypotensive and deteriorate rapidly.
2. The infant could remain in distress, despite ventilation, stimulation and rewarming, requiring a check for hypoglycemia or a more patent airway.
3. The mother could have a history (or not) of diabetes and could be hypoglycemic. She could also have a history of drug abuse (e.g. heroin) requiring naloxone for both the mother and the baby.
4. This baby could be the first of twins.
5. The mother could develop acute dyspnea from an amniotic embolus.
6. Any scene hazard can be incorporated, at the presenter's discretion. (This is in addition to or replacement of those already mentioned.)
7. Additional difficulty of airway management can be accomplished by adding vomiting to the scenario or by making the candidate have to intubate the mother.
8. The presenter may wish to make the infant more difficult to resuscitate (requiring intubation, drugs, and so on).
9. If deep tracheal suctioning is not completed, then the baby's condition should deteriorate rapidly.
10. Any location can be given to test the candidate's street or address competency, using local running cards.

SUMMARY

This mother is suffering from severe postpartum hemorrhage, leading to hypovolemic shock. The hemorrhage is not controlled despite fundal massage. The treatment would be the same as for any other hemorrhagic shock: oxygen, antishock garment, and IV fluid resuscitation. To complicate the scenario, the neonate is in distress, requiring the treatment of both patients. The neonate's primary problem is hypoxia. The birth has caused fetal distress through meconium aspiration. The meconium staining of the amniotic fluid is an ominous sign in itself. Meconium is a green, thick, tenacious fecal material defecated by the fetus during the delivery. The aspiration of the meconium requires vigorous airway suctioning. It may require direct laryngeal visualization and suctioning to assure that as much meconium as possible is removed. If the meconium reaches the level of the aveoli, it will interfere with gas exchange and cause severe hypoxia. Neonates primarily arrest from airway problems, not cardiac problems. Neonatal distress is usually indicated by bradycardia, not tachycardia. A heart rate of less than 100, in a neonate, is considered bradycardia. The first step to take, after suctioning, would be to ventilate with supplemental oxygen. Neonates are susceptible to hypothermia because of their greater surface area in relation to body mass, their immature thermoregulatory center, and their very limited amount of brown fat. The brown fat is used for energy to produce heat, as well as for insulation from heat loss, drying the amniotic fluid and blood from the neonate both stimulates the newborn and reduces the hypothermia. If the heart rate of the neonate drops below 80, CPR should be promptly initiated, following the American Heart Association infant guidelines.

OBSTETRICAL SCENARIO 4

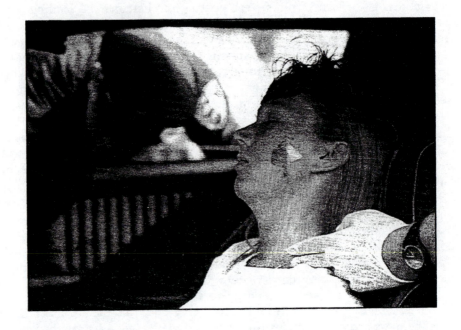

Type: Combination—obstetric, trauma.
Scenario moulage/prop list: Live model or mannequin, pillow, mortician's wax and plastic for impaled object in left cheek, simulated blood from nose, mouth, and ears, grease paint for pale skin color (motor vehicle setting).

INITIAL SCENE DESCRIPTION

Dispatch Information

LOCATION: Major intersection
NUMBER OF VICTIMS: Unknown
TYPE OF SITUATION: Auto accident with serious injuries
HAZARDS: Rush-hour traffic
WEATHER CONDITIONS: Cool and clear afternoon
TIME OF DAY: 1715 hours

Scene

You are dispatched through rush-hour traffic to an auto accident with "serious injuries." The police are on scene. While en route, the dispatcher informs you that PD has just called back and that "they have a woman who is pregnant and pulseless." When you arrive at the scene, you find total chaos and have trouble parking your vehicle due to the traffic. From across the way, you note that this is a one-car accident, car versus pole. It looks as though the patient can be easily extricated out the passenger side door. As you reach the patient, you note that she appears to have a massive head injury from striking the windshield, which is obviously indented. She is, in fact, apneic and pulseless. At that moment a police officer pulls you aside. He is looking at some papers he apparently found in the car. He says, "She just came from the doctor and she is 9 months pregnant."

PRIMARY ASSESSMENT FINDINGS

SCENE SURVEY

▾ major intersection

AIRWAY/CERVICAL SPINE

▾ airway open
▾ signs of trauma
▾ neck veins flat

BREATHING

▾ no breathing noted
▾ no chest rise

CIRCULATION/HEMORRHAGE CONTROL

▾ no carotid pulse
▾ no radial pulse
▾ capillary refill is immeasurable
▾ moderate amount of external blood from ears and nose
▾ large laceration to forehead

DISABILITY

▾ (A, V, P, U) unresponsive

EXPOSE AND EXAMINE

▾ piece of rearview mirror impaled in cheek
▾ obviously pregnant
▾ skin turgor good
▾ skin color pale
▾ skin warm and dry to touch
▾ weight estimated at 140 lb

SECONDARY ASSESSMENT FINDINGS

VITAL SIGNS

- respirations, 0
- pulse, 0
- blood pressure, 0
- ECG, asystole

HISTORY

- as above, except for the following:
  - A   unknown
  - M   prenatal care
  - P   full-term pregnancy
  - L   unknown
  - E   auto accident

HEAD

- large laceration to forehead
- depression and severe crepitus upon palpation
- bleeding and CFS noted from ears, nose, and mouth
- no Battle's signs, but raccoon's eyes present
- piece of rearview mirror impaled in cheek
- pupils dilated and nonreactive

NECK

- trachea midline
- neck veins flat
- no deformity
- no discoloration

CHEST

- no visible deformity
- no discoloration
- no chest wall movement
- no lung sounds
- no crepitus on palpation
- breast enlargement noted

ABDOMEN

- fundus is noted at the level of the xiphoid process
- abdomen distended with no contractions noted
- fetal heart tones present at a rate of 100
- external vaginal exam reveals no blood loss
- no crowning noted

EXTREMITIES

- ▾ obvious fracture right forearm
- ▾ no discoloration to others
- ▾ no visible signs of trauma to others
- ▾ capillary refill is immeasurable
- ▾ no distal pulses present
- ▾ skin turgor good
- ▾ skin warm and dry to touch
- ▾ tenderness, crepitus noted to right forearm
- ▾ no movement of extremities

NEUROLOGICAL

- ▾ unconscious, unresponsive
- ▾ Glascow coma scale calculated at 3:
    - ▾ eye opening, none (1)
    - ▾ verbal response, none (1)
    - ▾ motor response, none (1)

SENSORY EXAM

- ▾ unable to determine sensory or motor function

BACK

- ▾ no deformity
- ▾ no discoloration
- ▾ no trauma noted

Scenario Progression and Analysis: This scenario is a traumatic arrest and the patient cannot be saved. The baby she is carrying has a chance. The key to this scenario is rapid diagnosis, adequate CPR, and rapid transport to an appropriate facility. All BTLS/PHTLS interventions should be expedited on scene with the idea that CPR, with adequate oxygenation and volume, can keep the baby alive until a cesarean section is performed at the hospital.

SUGGESTED TREATMENT

EMT-A Level

- ▾ Conduct Scene Survey.
- ▾ Conduct Primary Assessment.
    - ▾ Remove impaled object from cheek.
- ▾ Suction vigorously.
    - ▾ Hyperventilate before and after.
    - ▾ Suction only on withdrawal.
    - ▾ Suction no longer than 10 seconds.

- ▾ Airway management should include proper application of the bag-valve-mask device with 100% O_2 administration.
  - ▾ Position patient properly with a pillow under her left hip.
  - ▾ Open airway with modified jaw thrust method.
  - ▾ Insert naso/oropharyngeal airway.
- ▾ Initiate proper CPR.
  - ▾ 5 to 1 ratio of compressions to ventilations.
  - ▾ 80 to 100 compressions per minute.
  - ▾ Proper hand placement and depth of compression.
- ▾ Conduct MAST survey and apply pneumatic antishock garment, legs only, as per local protocols.
- ▾ Reassess airway, breathing, and circulation.
- ▾ Transport ASAP.
- ▾ Conduct Secondary Assessment.
  - ▾ Dress bleeding areas and splint fractures.
- ▾ Notify appropriate receiving facility.
- ▾ Monitor fetal heart tones.

EMT-I Level

- ▾ Treatment is the same as above, but includes the following:
- ▾ Airway management should include insertion of an esophageal airway.
  - ▾ Place in sniffing position.
  - ▾ Assess lung sounds.
- ▾ Apply automatic external defibrillator, as per local protocols.
- ▾ Establish at least two large-bore IVs, infusing Ringer's lactate, open.
- ▾ Reassess airway, breathing, and circulation.

EMT-P Level

- ▾ Conduct Scene Survey.
- ▾ Conduct Primary Assessment, including rapid assessment of ECG, showing asystole.
  - ▾ Confirm in two leads.
  - ▾ Remove impaled object from cheek.
- ▾ Suction vigorously.
  - ▾ Hyperventilate before and after.
  - ▾ Suction only on withdrawal.
  - ▾ Suction no longer than 10 seconds.
- ▾ Airway management should include proper application of the bag-valve-mask device with 100% O_2 administration.
  - ▾ Position patient properly with a pillow under the left hip.
  - ▾ Open airway with modified jaw thrust method.
  - ▾ Insert naso/oropharyngeal airway.

- ▾ Initiate proper CPR.
    - ▾ 5 to 1 ratio of compressions to ventilations.
    - ▾ 80 to 100 compressions per minute
- ▾ Complete oral intubation with appropriate-sized tube.
    - ▾ Hyperventilate before and after.
    - ▾ No longer than 30 seconds.
    - ▾ Assess lung sounds.
- ▾ Conduct MAST survey and apply pneumatic antishock garment, legs only as per local protocols.
- ▾ Reassess airway, breathing, and circulation.
- ▾ Transport ASAP.
- ▾ Establish at least two large bore IVs, infusing Ringer's lactate, open.
- ▾ Reassess airway, breathing, and circulation.
- ▾ Notify appropriate receiving facility.
- ▾ Conduct Secondary Assessment.
    - ▾ Dress bleeding areas and splint fractures.
- ▾ Monitor fetal heart tones.
- ▾ Administer cardiac drug as per local protocols.

ADDITIONAL PROBLEMS

Depending on the level of the candidate, the following problems can be added to the scenario:

1. Despite adequate compressions, no palpable pulses are felt because of severe blood loss. (CPR should be continued anyway.)
2. Fetal heart rate may decrease even more, despite appropriate resuscitation efforts.
3. After removing the impaled object, bleeding may hamper airway management.
4. This baby could be delivered and be in arrest.
5. Any scene hazard can be incorporated at the presenter's discretion. (This is in addition to or replacement of those already mentioned.)
6. Any location can be given to test the candidate's street or address competency, using local running cards.
7. The patient's ECG rhythm could progress into a ventricular fibrillation.

SUMMARY

The candidate should recognize this is a load-and-go scenario. After the primary survey, the prehospital care provider should decide to minimally stabilize this patient on backboard and transport to the closest appropriate hospital. Airway and CPR are the priority. The female patient will not survive, but if the airway and CPR are preformed correctly and rapid transport is accomplished, an emergency cesarean section could save the yet unborn child. The emphasis is on recognition of the high mortality seen with traumatic asystole in blunt trauma. The candidates are not tested in this scenario on their resuscitative skills, but on the speed with which they identify that they cannot provide the definitive care that is needed to save the child's life. They should also recognize that the mother is not salvageable and all resuscitation efforts are directed toward saving her unborn child. Once the baby has been delivered, the resuscitation of the mother will be discontinued.

Chapter 4

PEDIATRIC SCENARIOS

PEDIATRIC SCENARIO 1

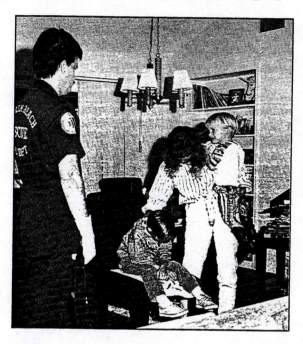

Type: Combination—pediatric, respiratory.
Scenario moulage/prop list: Live model or mannequin, live model
for mother's role, metaproterenol inhaler, grease paint for pale skin
color, glycerin water for skin (living-room setting).

INITIAL SCENE DESCRIPTION

Dispatch Information

LOCATION: Residential home
NUMBER OF VICTIMS: 1
TYPE OF SITUATION: Shortness of breath
HAZARDS: None
WEATHER CONDITIONS: Cloudy afternoon
TIME OF DAY: 1100 hours

Scene

You arrive at a house in the suburbs. A frantic woman meets you at the door as you get out of your truck. She says that her 5-year-old son is having an asthma attack and that "the inhaler is not working." After getting your equipment, the mother directs you to the boy, who is obviously in acute respiratory distress. He is leaning forward, not drooling, but gasping for air. The mother states she had him use his "inhaler" 5 times before she called 911.

PRIMARY ASSESSMENT FINDINGS

SCENE SURVEY

- ▼ residential home
- ▼ boy sitting in chair leaning forward
- ▼ a frantic mother

AIRWAY/CERVICAL SPINE

- ▼ airway open
- ▼ no signs of trauma
- ▼ neck veins flat

BREATHING

- ▼ 44 breaths per minute, labored
- ▼ limited but symmetrical chest wall rise
- ▼ lung sounds reveal occasional wheezing bilaterally
- ▼ lung sounds barely audible

CIRCULATION/HEMORRHAGE CONTROL

- ▼ regular, carotid pulse at 132
- ▼ regular radial, pulse at 132
- ▼ capillary refill at 3 seconds
- ▼ no obvious external blood loss

DISABILITY

- ▼ (A, V, P, U) alert but becoming sluggish

EXPOSE AND EXAMINE

- ▼ no obvious deformity or discoloration
- ▼ skin turgor good
- ▼ skin color pale

- ▾ skin cool and diaphoretic to touch
- ▾ weight estimated at 70 lb

SECONDARY ASSESSMENT FINDINGS

VITAL SIGNS

- ▾ respirations, 44 and labored
- ▾ pulse, 132 and regular
- ▾ blood pressure, 108/50
- ▾ ECG, a sinus tachycardia without ectopy

HISTORY

- ▾ as above, except for the following:
  - ▾ A   tetanus toxoid
  - ▾ M   metaproterenol
  - ▾ P   asthma
  - ▾ L   normal breakfast that morning, 2 hours ago
  - ▾ E - playing on his swing set

HEAD

- ▾ no visible trauma
- ▾ circumoral cyanosis noted
- ▾ no deformity on palpation
- ▾ pupils equal and reactive to light

NECK

- ▾ trachea midline
- ▾ neck veins flat
- ▾ exaggerated neck muscle use during inspiration
- ▾ no discoloration

CHEST

- ▾ no visible deformity
- ▾ no discoloration
- ▾ imited but symmetrical chest wall movement
- ▾ lung sounds reveal occasional wheezing bilaterally
- ▾ lung sounds barely audible
- ▾ intercostal muscle use during inspiration
- ▾ appears hyperinflated
- ▾ movement of extremities equal

ABDOMEN

- ▾ abdomen slightly distended
- ▾ soft, nontender to palpation
- ▾ (if checked, bowel sounds present)
- ▾ pelvic rock stable

EXTREMITIES

- ▾ no deformity
- ▾ cyanosis noted distally
- ▾ no visible signs of trauma
- ▾ capillary refill at 3 seconds
- ▾ distal pulses present
- ▾ skin turgor good
- ▾ skin cool and wet to touch
- ▾ no tenderness, crepitus, or swelling
- ▾ movement of extremities equal

NEUROLOGICAL

- ▾ conscious, alert but becoming progressively more sluggish
- ▾ Glascow coma scale calculated at 15:
  - ▾ eye opening, spontaneous (4)
  - ▾ verbal response, oriented (5)
  - ▾ motor response, obeys (5)

SENSORY EXAM

- ▾ no deficit in sensory or motor function

BACK

- ▾ no deformity
- ▾ no discoloration
- ▾ no trauma noted

Scenario Progression and Analysis: This patient is in acute respiratory dis tress due to status asthmaticus. EMT–As and Is should be tested on how quickly they diagnose the problem, properly control the airway and administer oxygen and transport or call for an ALS Unit. Paramedics should be tested on how quick ly they diagnose the problem, properly control the airway with high-flow oxy gen, and administer an aerosol treatment and/or epinephrine 1 : 1,000, subcuta neously. Midway through the scenario, the patient will go into respiratory and then cardiac arrest. If PALS guidelines are followed, this patient's condition will improve. If not, the boy's condition should deteriorate.

SUGGESTED TREATMENT

EMT-A Level

- Conduct Scene Survey.
  - Remove or calm the mother.
- Conduct Primary Assessment.
- Recognize this as a true respiratory emergency and transport rapidly or call for an ALS Unit.
- Airway management should include high-flow O_2 administration with a mask.
- Reassess airway, breathing, circulation, and level of consciousness.
- Conduct Secondary Assessment.

AT THIS TIME ,THE PATIENT BECOMES UNRESPONSIVE (APNEIC AND PULSELESS).

- Airway management should include proper application of the bag-valve-mask device with 100% O_2 administration.
  - Position patient properly.
  - Open airway with head-tilt, chin-lift.
  - Insert naso/oropharyngeal airway.
- Initiate proper CPR.
  - 5 to 1 ratio of compressions to ventilations.
  - 80 to 100 compressions per minute.
  - Proper hand placement and depth of compression (child).
- Reassess airway, breathing, circulation, and level of consciousness.
- Notify appropriate receiving facility.

EMT-I Level

- Treatment is the same as above, but includes the following:
- Airway management should not include insertion of an esophageal airway because of the patient's age and size.
- Establish a large-bore IV, infusing normal saline, as per local protocols, KVO.

EMT-P Level

- Conduct Scene Survey.
  - Remove or calm the mother.
- Conduct Primary Assessment.
- Airway management should include high-flow O_2 administration with a mask.

- Establish a large bore IV, infusing normal saline, as per local protocols, KVO.
- Conduct Secondary Assessment.
- Administer an aerosol treatment or 0.01 ml/kg of epinephrine, 1 :1 ,000, subcutaneously, as per local protocols.
- Reassess airway, breathing, circulation, and level of consciousness.

THE PATIENT REMAINS IN EXTREME RESPIRATORY DISTRESS (44 BREATHS/MINUTE).

- Repeat aerosol treatment and/or administer epinephrine, 0.01 ml/kg, subcutaneously, as per local protocols.
- Reassess airway, breathing, circulation, and level of consciousness.

AT THIS TIME, THE PATIENT BECOMES UNRESPONSIVE (APNEIC AND PULSELESS).

- Rapidly assess ECG, showing asystole.
  - Confirm in two leads.
- Airway management should include proper application of the bag-valve-mask device with 100%O_2 administration.
  - Position patient properly.
  - Open airway with head-tilt, chin-lift.
  - Insert naso/oropharyngeal airway.
- Initiate proper CPR.
  - 5 to 1 ratio of compressions to ventilations.
  - 80 to 100 compressions per minute
  - Proper hand placement and depth of compression (child).
- Complete oral intubation with appropriate-sized tube.
  - Hyperventilate before and after.
  - No longer than 30 seconds.
  - Assess lung sounds.
- Administer 0.01 mg/kg of epinephrine, 1 : 10,000, IV.
- Reassess ECG, airway, breathing, circulation, and level of consciousness.

ECG = SINUS TACHYCARDIA WITH A CORRESPONDING PULSE OF 128 BPM.

PATIENT IS STILL APNEIC.

BP = 78/40.

- Transport ASAP.
- Administer fluid bolus of 20 cc/kg of normal saline , as per local protocols.
- Reassess ECG airway, breathing, circulation, and level of consciousness.

▼ Notify appropriate receiving facility.

ADDITIONAL PROBLEMS

Depending on the level of the candidate, the following problems can be added to the scenario:

1. The candidate may have difficulty with an IV, since the patient is only five years old.
2. The presenter may wish to make the patient's ECG go from asystole to bradycardia, instead of a sinus tachycardia.
3. The candidate may have difficulty with oral intubation.
4. Following the administration of the aerosol, or epinephrine, the patient may experience an atrial tachycardia with a rapid ventricular response.
5. If an esophageal airway is inserted, the patient will rapidly deteriorate into cardiac arrest.
6. When first assessing the patient, the candidate may not hear lung sounds. The reason for this is that, since the patient's lungs are so tight, no air is moving during ventilation.
7. Any scene hazard can be incorporated at the presenter's discretion. (This is in addition to or replacement of those already mentioned.)
8. The presenter may wish to take the candidate further down the asystolic algorithm before allowing the patient to come out.
9. If the airway is not aggressively managed, the patient can deteriorate even more rapidly.
10. Any location can be given to test the candidate's street or address competency, using local running cards.
11. If a pulse oximeter reading is asked for by the candidate, an appropriate reading should be given.
12. During airway management, the endotracheal tube placement can take too long or be improperly placed in the right bronchus.

SUMMARY

This child suffers from asthma. The assessment of the pediatric patient is complicated by the age of the child and the difficulty in obtaining history. The physical assessment may be difficult because the child is not cooperative. Many times the assessment can begin at the door. If the child is listless and not active, then he or she needs your intervention. If the child can fight the caregiver, then, more than likely, he or she is stable. In the child with asthma, the absence of lung sounds is an ominous sign. The airway is so hyperinflated and constricted that the patient cannot move adequate tidal volumes; intervention is required immediately. Children with asthma may also become tolerant to the prehospital drugs routinely used to treat asthma. Consequently, they may not respond to the treatment and deteriorate rapidly.

The prehospital provider must remember that airway management may not always include the use of an esophageal airway; it is, of course, contraindicated for use in children under 15 years of age. Due to the size of a child's esophagus, the EOA would be too long and not seal it, distally. BLS must be adjusted for the size of the child with proper hand placement and depth of compressions. The primary cause of cardiac arrest in children is not cardiac in origin. The usual causes are respiratory. Vigorous airway management and high concentrations of O_2 are the most beneficial treatments. If drug therapy is indicated in arrest situations, epinephrine is the first-line drug. Problems with children are not usually cardiovascular in nature as seen in adults. Ventricular fibrillation is rarely seen in children; asystole and bradycardia are more likely to occur.

PEDIATRIC SCENARIO 2

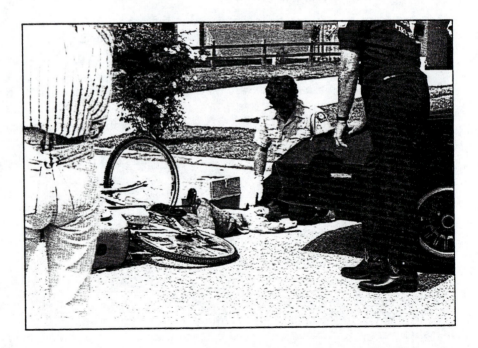

Type: Combination—trauma, pediatric.
Scenario moulage/prop list: Live child model or mannequin live model as police role, live models as bystanders, bicycle, grease paint for pale skin color and contusion left temple and left chest, glycerin water for skin (street setting).

INITIAL SCENE DESCRIPTION

Dispatch Information

LOCATION: Residential street
NUMBER OF VICTIMS: Unknown
TYPE OF SITUATION: Child hit by car
HAZARDS: Traffic
WEATHER CONDITIONS: Warm, clear morning
TIME OF DAY: 1003

Scene

You are at a local car wash when an alarm comes in as a "child hit by car." It's not your call, but you are the closest unit, so you cancel the other rescue truck and respond. You see that a crowd has formed, and your partner quickly heads to the scene as you hustle to get the equipment. A police officer directs you to the boy who was on the bicycle, saying, "Only the boy was hurt." You find a 7-year-old male lying left laterally recumbent next to an oversized bike, with obvious bruising to his left temporal area and left thoracic region. He is responsive only to painful stimuli and his capillary refill is 4 seconds.

PRIMARY ASSESSMENT FINDINGS

SCENE SURVEY

- residential street
- child left laterally recumbent on road
- possible traffic hazard

AIRWAY/CERVICAL SPINE

- open airway
- signs of trauma
- neck veins flat

BREATHING

- 32 breaths per minute, shallow
- unequal chest rise noted
- lung sounds diminished on left

CIRCULATION/HEMORRHAGE CONTROL

- rapid, weak carotid pulse at 128
- rapid, weak radial pulse at 128

- ▼ capillary refill delayed to 4 seconds
- ▼ no obvious external blood loss

DISABILITY

- ▼ (A, V, P, U) combatively responds to pain

EXPOSE AND EXAMINE

- ▼ contusion noted to left temple
- ▼ contusion noted to left side of chest
- ▼ skin turgor good
- ▼ skin color pale
- ▼ skin cool and diaphoretic to touch
- ▼ weight estimated at 60 lb

SECONDARY ASSESSMENT FINDINGS

VITAL SIGNS

- ▼ respirations, 32 and shallow
- ▼ pulse, 128
- ▼ blood pressure, 100/60
- ▼ ECG, a sinus tachycardia

HISTORY

- ▼ as above, except for the following:
    - ▼ A   unknown
    - ▼ M   unknown
    - ▼ P   unknown
    - ▼ L   unknown
    - ▼ E   riding bike

HEAD

- ▼ contusion to left temple
- ▼ crepitus on palpation of left temple
- ▼ no Battle's signs or raccoon's eyes
- ▼ pupils midrange and reactive to light

NECK

- ▼ trachea midline
- ▼ neck veins flat
- ▼ no deformity
- ▼ no discoloration

CHEST

- ▼ contusion noted to left chest area
- ▼ paradoxical left chest wall motion
- ▼ diminished lung sounds on left
- ▼ crepitus noted on left to several ribs
- ▼ dull upon percassion on left
- ▼ tenderness on palpation to same area

ABDOMEN

- ▼ abdomen nondistended
- ▼ soft, nontender to palpation
- ▼ (if checked, bowel sounds present)
- ▼ pelvic rock unstable with crepitus

EXTREMITIES

- ▼ no deformity
- ▼ no discoloration
- ▼ no visible signs of trauma
- ▼ capillary refill delayed to 4 seconds
- ▼ rapid, weak distal pulses present
- ▼ skin color pale
- ▼ skin turgor good
- ▼ skin cool and diaphoretic to touch
- ▼ no tenderness, crepitus, or swelling noted
- ▼ movement of extremities equal

NEUROLOGICAL

- ▼ obtunded, responsive to pain
- ▼ Glascow coma scale calculated at 7:
    - ▼ eye opening, none (1)
    - ▼ verbal response, incomprehensible sounds (2)
    - ▼ motor response, withdraws but with some spontaneous movement (4)

PEDIATRIC TRAUMA SCORE: 7

- ▼ weight, +2
- ▼ airway, -1
- ▼ BP, +2
- ▼ LOC, +1
- ▼ open wound, +2
- ▼ fractures, +1

▼ combative in response to painful stimuli

BACK

▼ no deformity
▼ no discoloration
▼ no trauma noted

Scenario Progression and Analysis: This is a trauma scenario with four major problems. The boy has a head injury, a hemothorax combined with a flail chest, and is suffering from hypovolemia due to hemorrhagic shock from a fractured pelvic. EMT–As, Is, and paramedics should all be tested on rapid diagnosis of the problems, proper airway control, cervical-spine immobilization, stabilization of the flail section, antishock garment application (as per local protocols), and the decision to transport ASAP or call for ALS assistance. EMT–Is and paramedics should also be tested on their volume replacement. Midway through the scenario, this patient will go into cardiac arrest.

SUGGESTED TREATMENT

EMT-A Level

▼ Conduct Scene Survey.
  ▼ Have police control scene.
▼ Conduct Primary Assessment.
▼ Airway management should include proper application of the bag-valve-mask device with 100% O_2 administration.
  ▼ Position patient properly.
  ▼ Open airway with modified jaw thrust method.
  ▼ Insert oropharyngeal airway.
  ▼ Continue to hyperventilate patient.
▼ Maintain cervical spine manually during and after airway management.
▼ Stabilize flail segment, as per local protocols.
▼ Reassess airway, breathing, circulation, and level of consciousness.
▼ Secure patient with cervical immobilization devices to backboard.
▼ Consider elevation of the head of the backboard 15 degrees to help decrease intracranial pressure once capillary refill has improved.
▼ Conduct MAST survey and apply pneumatic antishock garment, as per local protocols.
▼ Reassess airway, breathing, circulation, and level of consciousness.

**AT THIS TIME, THE PATIENT BECOMES APNEIC
AND PULSELESS.**

- Initiate proper CPR.
  - 5 to 1 ratio of compressions to ventilations.
  - 80 to100 compressions per minute.
  - Proper hand placement and depth of compression (child).
- Transport ASAP or call for an ALS Unit.
- Notify appropriate receiving facility.
- Conduct Secondary Assessment.

EMT-I Level

- Treatment is the same as above, but includes the following:
- Airway management should *not* include insertion of an esophageal airway.
- Establish at least one large-bore IV of 0.9% normal saline or Ringer's lactate, infusing 20 cc/kg.
  - Repeat, as needed.
- Reassess airway, breathing, circulation, and level of consciousness.

EMT-P Level

- Conduct Scene Survey.
  - Have police control scene.
- Conduct Primary Assessment.
- Airway management should include proper application of the bag-valve-mask device with 100% O_2 administration.
  - Position patient properly.
  - Open airway with modified jaw thrust method.
  - Insert oropharyngeal airway.
- Maintain cervical spine manually during and after airway management.
- Stabilize flail segment, as per local protocols.
- Reassess airway, breathing, circulation, and level of consciousness.
- Complete oral intubation with appropriate-sized tube.
  - Hyperventilate before and after.
  - No longer than 30 seconds.
  - Assess lung sounds.
  - Continue to hyperventilate patient .
- Consider elevation of the head of the backboard 15 degrees to help decrease intracranial pressure once capillary refill has improved.
- Conduct MAST survey and apply pneumatic antishock garment, as per local protocols.
- Reassess airway, breathing, circulation, and level of consciousness.

AT THIS TIME, THE PATIENT BECOMES APNEIC AND PULSELESS.

- ▼ Initiate proper CPR.
  - ▼ 5 to 1 ratio of compressions to ventilations.
  - ▼ 80 to100 compressions per minute.
  - ▼ Proper hand placement and depth of compression (child).
- ▼ Assess ECG rapidly, showing asystole.
  - ▼ Confirm in two leads.
- ▼ Transport ASAP.
- ▼ Establish at least one large-bore IV of normal saline or Ringer's lactate, infusing 20 cc/kg.
  - ▼ Repeat, as needed.
- ▼ Reassess ECG, airway, breathing, circulation, and level of consciousness.
- ▼ Administer epinephrine and atropine as per PALS guidelines or as per local protocols.
- ▼ Notify appropriate receiving facility.
- ▼ Conduct Secondary Assessment.

ADDITIONAL PROBLEMS

Depending on the level of the candidate, the following problems can be added to the scenario:

1. Due to the fact that this is a child, IV access may be unavailable, requiring an intraosseous infusion.
2. Endotracheal intubation may be made more difficult so that the candidate may have to make the decision to stay on scene.
3. Any history (such as diabetes) can be given initially, but the proper treatment for the history should be followed during the arrest (that is, blood drawn, 50% dextrose given).
4. Fractures of extremities could be given so that more splinting would eventually be required by the candidate.
5. Any location can be given to test the candidate's street or address competency, using local running cards.
6. Any scene hazard can be incorporated at the presenter's discretion. (This is in addition to or replacement of those already mentioned.)
7. During the scenario, make CPR ineffective and require depth change.
8. If universal precautions are not followed, the candidate can be told, after the scenario, that the patient had HIV or hepatitis.

SUMMARY

Any time the prehospital care provider is faced with an injured child, the stress increases. Trauma care is stressful by itself, but when the trauma is a child, it becomes even more difficult. The care of the pediatric patient is not like that of the adult, since they are smaller and have better reserves. They compensate well during early stages of shock and injury; they also deteriorate rapidly once the compensatory mechanisms begin to fail. Luckily, the prehospital care provider is not frequently presented with situations dealing with pediatric trauma. But the required knowledge and skills, since treatment differs from that of the adult, can deteriorate rapidly if not frequently rehearsed or used. The devices normally used for treatment of the trauma patient may not fit the pediatric patient. Properly sized devices should be available and utilized during this scenario.

Traumatic arrest treatment should be directed at the cause of the arrest. In most cases the team is made up of only two or three providers. If three are available, one should deal with the airway and cervical spine. The second should perform cardiac compressions, and the third should perform a primary survey. During the primary survey, any life-threatening problems should be treated. In this scenario, the flail segment will interfere with the mechanics of ventilation. Early recognition and stabilization are required. Drug therapy in trauma arrests should not be forgotten, although volume infusion should be accomplished first. Once this is done, ACLS guidelines should be followed; however, it must be realized that rapid transport to an appropriate facility should be the priority.

PEDIATRIC SCENARIO 3

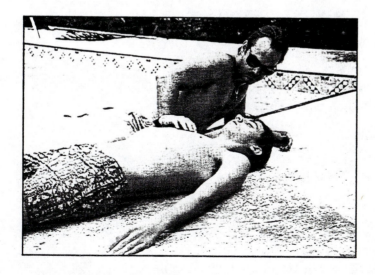

Type: Combination—trauma, pediatric.
Scenario moulage/prop list: Live model or mannequin, live model for lifeguard's role, backboard, grease paint for pale skin color, glycerin water for skin (pool setting).

INITIAL SCENE DESCRIPTION

Dispatch Information

LOCATION: Local municipal pool
NUMBER OF VICTIMS: 1
TYPE OF SITUATION: Water injury
HAZARDS: None
WEATHER CONDITIONS: Warm, sunny afternoon
TIME OF DAY: 1325 hours

Scene

You arrive on scene at a local municipal park and are quickly directed to the pool area by one of the lifeguards. He explains the situation, as you remove all your needed equipment from the truck. It seems that a rather large 14 year old was "horsing around" and dived into the shallow end of the pool. Shortly after the dive, he was found unconscious by one of the pool guards. The lifeguard continues, "We got him out of the pool with a backboard as soon as we could...he is breathing." You arrive to find the large, young male beside the pool, supine on a backboard, with no other devices applied to him. The guard states he does not think that his parents will arrive to pick him up for at least another hour.

PRIMARY ASSESSMENT FINDINGS

SCENE SURVEY

- ▼ municipal pool
- ▼ boy supine on backboard
- ▼ no apparent hazards

AIRWAY/CERVICAL SPINE

- ▼ airway open
- ▼ neck veins flat

BREATHING

- ▼ 32 breaths per minute, shallow
- ▼ symmetrical chest rise
- ▼ lung sounds clear bilaterally

CIRCULATION/HEMORRHAGE CONTROL

- ▼ regular carotid pulse at 64
- ▼ no radial pulse

- capillary refill delayed to 5 seconds
- no obvious external blood loss

DISABILITY

- (A, V, P, U) unresponsive

EXPOSE AND EXAMINE

- large hematoma to mid-forehead
- skin turgor good
- skin color pale
- skin warm and wet to touch
- weight estimated at 200 lb

SECONDARY ASSESSMENT FINDINGS

VITAL SIGNS

- respirations, 32 and shallow
- pulse, 64 and regular
- blood pressure, 70/50
- ECG, a normal sinus rhythm

HISTORY

- as above, except for the following:
  - A   unknown
  - M   unknown
  - P   diabetes
  - L   unknown
  - E   dove into shallow end of pool

HEAD

- large hematoma to mid-forehead
- crepitus to area on palpation
- no other visible trauma
- pupils equal and reactive
- no CSF noted
- no Battle's signs or raccoon's eyes

NECK

- trachea midline
- neck veins flat

- ▼ deformity noted to the upper back of the neck
- ▼ slight discoloration noted in the area of deformity
- ▼ medical alert tag on a necklace—"diabetes"

CHEST

- ▼ no visible deformity
- ▼ no discoloration
- ▼ slight but symmetrical chest wall movement
- ▼ abdominal breathing noted
- ▼ lung sounds clear and equal
- ▼ no deformity, tenderness, or crepitus on palpation

ABDOMEN

- ▼ abdomen nondistended
- ▼ soft, nontender to palpation
- ▼ (if checked, bowel sounds present)
- ▼ priapism present
- ▼ pelvic rock stable

EXTREMITIES

- ▼ no deformity
- ▼ no discoloration
- ▼ no visible signs of trauma
- ▼ capillary refill delayed to 5 seconds
- ▼ no distal pulses present
- ▼ skin turgor good
- ▼ skin color pale
- ▼ skin warm and wet to touch
- ▼ no tenderness, crepitus, or swelling
- ▼ no spontaneous movement of extremities

NEUROLOGICAL

- ▼ unconscious, unresponsive
- ▼ Glasgow coma scale calculated at 3:
    - ▼ eye opening, none (1)
    - ▼ verbal response, none (1)
    - ▼ motor response, none (1)

SENSORY EXAM

- ▼ unable to determine sensory or motor function

BACK

- ▾ deformity palpated to upper neck
- ▾ slight discoloration to same area
- ▾ no crepitus noted

Scenario Progression and Analysis: This patient has had a C5/C6 cervical fracture, which has severed his spinal cord. The emphasis should be placed on nonmanipulation of the patient with proper airway control, appropriate spinal immobilization, and treatment for the neurogenic shock. EMT-As and Is should be tested on how quickly they diagnose the problem, initiate proper airway management, secure the patient, apply the pneumatic antishock garment and transport or call for ALS assistance. Paramedics should be tested on how quickly they diagnose the cord injury, properly control the airway, hyperventilate, and initiate treatment, including volume replacement and then administer dopamine to increase the blood pressure of the patient. If the diagnosis and treatment are completed rapidly, the patient's condition will improve. If BTLS/PHTLS guidelines are not followed, this patient should either remain the same or deteriorate.

SUGGESTED TREATMENT

EMT-A Level

- ▾ Conduct Scene Survey.
- ▾ Conduct Primary Assessment.
- ▾ Airway management should include proper application of the bag-valve-mask device with 100% O_2 administration.
    - ▾ Position patient properly.
    - ▾ Open airway with modified jaw thrust method.
    - ▾ Insert oropharyngeal airway.
- ▾ Reassess airway, breathing, circulation, and level of consciousness.
- ▾ Maintain cervical spine manually, during and after airway management.
- ▾ Secure patient with cervical immobilization devices to backboard.

AT THIS TIME, THE PATIENT VOMITS.

- ▾ Suction vigorously.
    - ▾ Hyperventilate before and after.
    - ▾ Suction only on withdrawal.
    - ▾ Suction no longer than 10 seconds.
- ▾ Reassess airway, breathing, circulation, and level of consciousness.
- ▾ Conduct MAST survey.
- ▾ Cover patient to prevent further heat loss.

- Apply pneumatic antishock garment, as per local protocols.
- Reassess airway, breathing, circulation, and level of consciousness.

PATIENT'S LEVEL OF CONSCIOUSNESS REMAINS THE SAME. PATIENT'S CAPILLARY REFILL= 3 SECONDS. PATIENT'S BP = 98/58.

- Transport ASAP or call for an ALS Unit.
- Consider elevation of the head of the backboard 15 degrees to help decrease intracranial pressure.
- Reassess airway, breathing, circulation, and level of consciousness
- Conduct Secondary Assessment.
- Notify appropriate receiving facility.

EMT-I Level

- Treatment is the same as above, but includes the following:
- Airway management should *not* include insertion of an esophageal airway because of the patient's age and size.
- Establish two large-bore IVs infusing Ringer's lactate or normal saline, open.
- Reassess airway, breathing, circulation, and level of consciousness.

PATIENT'S LEVEL OF CONSCIOUSNESS REMAINS THE SAME. PATIENT'S CAPILLARY REFILL = 3 SECONDS. PATIENT'S BP = 108/68.

EMT-P Level

- Conduct Scene Survey.
- Conduct Primary Assessment, which includes rapid assessment of ECG, showing a normal sinus rhythm.
- Airway management should include proper application of the bag-valve-mask device with 100% O_2 administration.
    - Position patient properly.
    - Open airway with modified jaw thrust method.
    - Insert oropharyngeal airway.
    - Continue to hyperventilate patient.
- Reassess ECG, airway, breathing, circulation ,and level of consciousness.
- Maintain cervical spine manually, during and after airway management.
- Secure patient with cervical immobilization devices to backboard.

AT THIS TIME, THE PATIENT VOMITS.

- Suction vigorously.
  - Hyperventilate before and after.
  - Suction only on withdrawal.
  - Suction no longer than 10 seconds.
- Complete oral intubation with appropriate-sized tube.
  - Hyperventilate before and after.
  - No longer than 30 seconds.
  - Assess lung sounds.
  - Continue to hyperventilate patient .
- Conduct MAST survey.
- Cover patient to prevent further heat loss.
- Apply pneumatic antishock garment, as per local protocols.
- Reassess ECG, airway, breathing, circulation, and level of consciousness.

NO CHANGE IN THE STATUS OF THE PATIENT.

- Transport ASAP.
- Draw blood sample and obtain glucometer/glucostrip reading.
- Establish two large-bore IVs infusing Ringer's lactate or normal saline, open.
- Reassess airway, breathing, circulation, and level of consciousness.

GLUCOSE READING = 120 MG/DL. NO CHANGE IN THE STATUS OF THE PATIENT.

- Consider administering naloxone, 2 mg (or 0.01 mg/kg), or as per local protocols.
- Reassess airway, breathing, circulation, and level of consciousness.
- Conduct Secondary Assessment.

PATIENT'S CAPILLARY REFILL = 4 SECONDS. PATIENTS BP= 70/50.

- Administer dopamine, as per local protocols.
- Reassess ECG, airway, breathing, circulation, and level of consciousness.

PATIENT'S LEVEL OF CONSCIOUSNESS REMAINS THE SAME. PATIENT'S CAPILLARY REFILL= 3 SECONDS. PATIENT'S BP = 90/60.

- Consider elevation of the head of the backboard 15 degrees to help decrease intracranial pressure.
- Reassess ECG, airway, breathing, circulation, and level of consciousness.
- Notify appropriate receiving facility.

ADDITIONAL PROBLEMS

Depending on the level of the candidate, the following problems can be added to the scenario:

1. The patient's airway may be made more difficult to manage by having the patient continue to vomit and not allow intubation.
2. Even though the history is directed toward trauma, the patient could respond to treatment for unknown origin because of narcotics or hypoglycemia.
3. Once backboarded, the patient may again vomit or experience a seizure.
4. Because of peripheral vasodilation and water immersion, the patient can present with mild hypothermia requiring re-warming.
5. If the patient's cervical spine is manipulated or ignored, the patient could go into respiratory arrest and subsequent cardiac arrest.
6. The addition of any scene hazard can be incorporated at the presenter's discretion. (This is in addition to or replacement of those already mentioned.)
7. Even after the proper treatment has been accomplished, the patient can still deteriorate and go into cardiac arrest to further test the candidate's knowledge.
8. The dopamine infusion could cause ectopy, requiring the proper intervention.
9. Any location can be given to test the candidate's street or address competency, using local running cards.

SUMMARY

When called to any shallow-water medical scene, a cervical spine injury should be suspected. The signs of hypotension, with an absence of tachycardia, indicate a high cord injury and neurogenic shock. Because of the separation of the cord, no stimulation to the autonomic nervous system can occur. This leads to a loss of vascular tone, hypotension, and a lack of compensatory tachycardia. The area of the cervical spine that is injured in this patient is at cervical vertebrae 5 and 6. The two most commonly injured areas in the cervical spine are C1 to 2 and C5 to 6. The presence of abdominal breathing suggests a lower-cervical-injury, a C5 to 6 problem. Because of vasodilation and enhanced heat loss, as well as being immersed in a pool, the neurogenic shock patient is extremely susceptible to hypothermia.

Treatment for neurogenic shock is initially directed toward volume expansion by way of pneumatic antishock garment application and then rapid infusion of IV fluids. But, because this is primarily a "container size" problem, dopamine can be effective by increasing cardiac output and limiting vasodilation. The prehospital care provider should treat this patient's cervical spine with extreme care. The cord may have already been severed, but further injury must be avoided.

When dealing with airway control, the head and neck should be manually stabilized: no cervical stabilization device, by itself, is sufficient. The combination of manual stabilization and a cervical collar will provide adequate protection from further injury, until immobilization with a long spine board can be accomplished.

PEDIATRIC SCENARIO 4

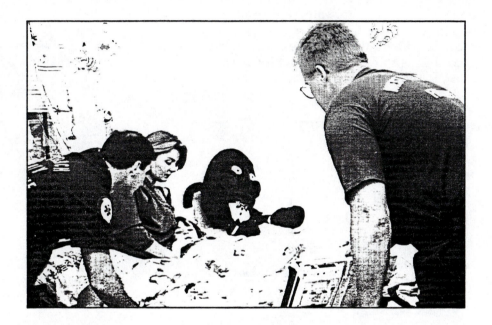

Type: Combination—medical, pediatric.
Scenario moulage/prop list: Live child model or mannequin, live model for hysterical mother, rouge for flushed skin color, glycerin water for skin, red or purple felt-tip marker for rash (bedroom setting).

INITIAL SCENE DESCRIPTION

Dispatch Information

LOCATION: Rural farmhouse
NUMBER OF VICTIMS: 1
TYPE OF SITUATION: Child with convulsions
HAZARDS: None apparent
WEATHER CONDITIONS: Clear, afternoon
TIME OF DAY: 1400 hours

Scene

You are called to a rural farmhouse where a 4-year-old female child is having seizures. After arriving, you enter the house to find the child awake, but disoriented to person, place, and time. She has been incontinent of urine sometime during the afternoon. The child's mother states that Ginny "has had a fever, on and off, for the last 3 days." Mom also explains that this morning she had complained of a severe headache and then, right before she called 911, Ginny appeared to have a seizure. You question Mom about any medications she may have given and she states that Ginny had some acetaminophen for the fever 2 hours before. As you begin your primary survey, the child's level of consciousness rapidly decreases and she begins to have generalized seizure activity for 30 seconds. The mother becomes extremely upset and begins to cry hysterically. Once the seizure stops, the child begins breathing, again very rapidly, but remains unconscious.

PRIMARY ASSESSMENT FINDINGS

SCENE SURVEY

- ▼ rural farmhouse, well kept
- ▼ hysterical mother in bedroom
- ▼ child supine in bed

AIRWAY/CERVICAL SPINE

- ▼ airway open, complicated by salivation
- ▼ no signs of trauma
- ▼ neck veins flat

BREATHING

- ▼ 28 breaths per minute, deep and snoring respirations
- ▼ symmetrical chest rise
- ▼ lungs clear bilaterally

CIRCULATION/HEMORRHAGE CONTROL

- ▼ rapid, bounding carotid pulse at 120
- ▼ rapid, strong radial pulse at 120
- ▼ capillary refill at 2 seconds
- ▼ no obvious external blood loss

DISABILITY

- ▼ (A, V, P, U) unconscious, responds to painful stimuli

EXPOSE AND EXAMINE

- ▼ no obvious deformity or discoloration
- ▼ skin color flushed
- ▼ skin turgor fair
- ▼ skin hot and diaphoretic to touch
- ▼ rash noted on upper chest
- ▼ weight estimated at 50 lb

SECONDARY ASSESSMENT FINDINGS

VITAL SIGNS

- ▼ respirations, 28 and snoring
- ▼ pulse, 120
- ▼ blood pressure, 100/70
- ▼ temperature, 102 degrees, axillary
- ▼ ECG, a sinus tachycardia

HISTORY

- ▼ as above, except for the following:
    - ▼ A   none
    - ▼ M   acetaminophen 2 hours prior with proper dose
    - ▼ P   normal childhood illnesses, fever for 3 days, severe headache this A.M., no history of seizures
    - ▼ L   cereal for breakfast
    - ▼ E   seizure activity 2 times

HEAD

- ▼ no visible trauma
- ▼ no deformity on palpation
- ▼ pupils equal and reactive to light
- ▼ no CSF noted
- ▼ no Battle's signs or raccoon's eyes

NECK

- ▼ trachea midline
- ▼ neck veins flat
- ▼ no deformity
- ▼ no discoloration
- ▼ (if checked, neck notably stiff)

CHEST

▼ petechial rash noted on upper chest wall
▼ symmetrical chest wall movement
▼ lung sounds clear and equal bilaterally
▼ no deformity, tenderness ,or crepitus on palpation

ABDOMEN

▼ abdomen nondistended
▼ soft, nontender to palpation
▼ (if checked, bowel sounds present)
▼ pelvic rock stable

EXTREMITIES

▼ no deformity
▼ no discoloration
▼ no visible signs of trauma
▼ capillary refill at 2 seconds
▼ bounding, rapid distal pulses present
▼ skin turgor fair
▼ skin color flushed
▼ skin hot and diaphoretic to touch
▼ no tenderness, crepitus, or swelling
▼ movement of all extremities equal

NEUROLOGICAL

▼ unconscious, responds only to painful stimuli
▼ Glascow coma scale calculated at 8:
  ▼ eye, opening to pain (2)
  ▼ verbal response, none (1)
  ▼ motor response, localizes (5)

SENSORY EXAM

▼ localizes painful stimuli and moves all extremities

BACK

▼ no deformity
▼ no discoloration
▼ rigidity noted

Scenario Progression and Analysis: The patient's level of consciousness continues to decrease into unresponsiveness. For EMT—As and Is, the seizure activity increases in frequency and duration if the fever is not treated with cooling (sponge bath with room temperature water is recommended). They should be tested on rapid recognition of the problem and how quickly they decide to transport or call for an ALS Unit. For the paramedics, the patient should deteriorate if diazepam is not administered. Due to the infectious nature of the findings, the importance of the proper protection of all involved (with masks, gloves, and the like) cannot be stressed enough.

SUGGESTED TREATMENT

EMT-A Level

- ▼ Conduct Scene Survey.
  - ▼ Remove or calm mother.
  - ▼ Use universal precautions for infection control.
- ▼ Conduct Primary Assessment.
- ▼ Suction vigorously.
  - ▼ Hyperventilate before and after.
  - ▼ Suction only on withdrawal.
  - ▼ Suction no longer than 10 seconds.
- ▼ Airway management should include proper application of the bag-valve-mask device with 100% O_2 administration.
  - ▼ Position patient properly.
  - ▼ Open airway with head-tilt, chin-lift.
  - ▼ Insert naso/oropharyngeal airway.

AT THIS TIME, THE PATIENT HAS A GRAND MAL SEIZURE.

- ▼ Protect patient's body from sharp objects.
- ▼ Remove patient's clothes and cool patient, as per local protocols.

THE PATIENT STOPS SEIZING.

- ▼ Reassess airway, breathing, circulation, and level of consciousness.
- ▼ Transport ASAP or call for an ALS Unit.
- ▼ Conduct Secondary Assessment.
- ▼ Notify appropriate receiving facility.

EMT-I Level

- ▼ Treatment is the same as above, but includes the following:
- ▼ Establish a large-bore IV infusing normal saline, as per local protocols, KVO.

EMT-P Level

- Conduct Scene Survey.
  - Remove or calm mother.
  - Use universal precautions for infection control.
- Conduct Primary Assessment, which includes a rapid assessment of ECG, showing a sinus tachycardia.
- Suction vigorously.
  - Hyperventilate before and after.
  - Suction only on withdrawal.
  - Suction no longer than 10 seconds.
- Airway management should include proper application of the bag-valve-mask device with 100% O_2 administration.
  - Position patient properly.
  - Open airway with head-tilt, chin-lift.
  - Insert naso/oropharyngeal airway.
- Complete oral intubation with appropriate-sized tube.
  - Hyperventilate before and after.
  - No longer than 30 seconds.
  - Assess lung sounds.

AT THIS TIME, THE PATIENT HAS A GRAND MAL SEIZURE.

- Continue to hyperventilate patient.
- Administer diazepam, ET, IM, or rectally. (If ET route is used, new ACLS guidelines suggest the medication should be increased to ten times the IV dose to assure absorbtion.)
- Protect patient's body from sharp objects.
- Remove patient's clothes and cool, as per local protocols.

THE PATIENT STOPS SEIZING.

- Reassess airway, breathing, circulation, and level of consciousness.

PATIENT'S LEVEL OF CONSCIOUSNESS DOES NOT CHANGE.

- Draw blood and obtain glucometer/glucostrip reading.

GLUCOSE READING = 82 MG/DL.

- Establish a large IV of normal saline, as per local protocols, KVO.
- Consider 0.01 mg/kg of naxolone, as per local protocols.
- Conduct Secondary Assessment.

▼ Transport ASAP.

▼ Notify appropriate receiving facility.

ADDITIONAL PROBLEMS

Depending on the level of the candidate, the following problems can be added to the scenario:

1. If universal precautions for protection are not followed, team members will be exposed to infectious meningitis.
2. The mother's care must be addressed, but ,if not, she should become so distraught that she interrupts the treatment.
3. Another problem for airway control during the seizure activity, like jaw clenching, could be added, requiring nasal intubation.
4. A delay in transport can also be added to this scenario to increase its difficulty.
5. Seizure activity should increase if the fever is not addressed.
6. The patient can go into respiratory arrest after the diazepam.
7. The patient can have another seizure requiring more diazepam.
8. Any location can be given to test the candidate's street or address competency, using local running cards.
9. Any scene hazard can be incorporated at the presenter's discretion. (This is in addition to or replacement of those already mentioned.)
10. A drug overdose or diabetic history can be included so that the candidate will have to address these problems with naloxone and 25% dextrose.

SUMMARY

This patient is suffering from meningococcal meningitis. This infection is of greatest risk to young children less than 10 years of age. Prehospital care providers can be at some risk of infection if universal precautions of protection are not followed with these types of patients. The infectious agent that causes this type of meningitis is *Neisseria meningitidis*. This organism lives in the nasopharynx and may enter the brain through the subarachnoid space, causing meningitis. The most common signs and symptoms of this type of infection include fever, nausea, stiff neck, headache, vomiting, and a rash (petechial) that appears on the body. Petechia are painless pinpoint lesions. The patient may also suffer a change in level of consciousness and seizures. Seizure activity can also be precipitated by high fevers. The hysterical mother should be removed, during the child's treatment, to facilitate a safe and cooperative environment.

The proper treatment includes proper airway management with oxygenation, cooling, and administration of diazepam when seizures persist (in this instance down the endotracheal tube).[7] Again, a room temperature sponge bath is recommended for cooling. Other types (alcohol, ice baths and wet sheets) are ineffective in reducing temperature and may actually have the reverse effect, by cooling peripherally and not centrally, causing shivering. Acetaminophen is most effective in reducing a fever of this type.

[7]"Guidelines for Cardiopulmonary Resuscitation and Emergency Care," JAMA, 268 (1992), No. 16, 2170-2298.

W.G. Barsan and others, "Blood Levels of Diazepam after Endotracheal Administration in Dogs," Emerg. Med. 11 (1982), 242-47.

Chapter 5

TOXICOLOGICAL SCENARIOS

TOXICOLOGICAL SCENARIO 1

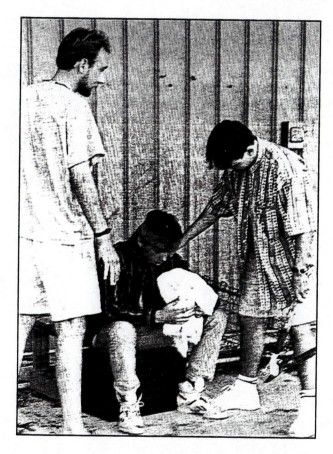

Type: Toxicological (ingestion of poison).
Scenario moulage/prop list: Live model or mannequin, several bystanders, grease paint for pale skin color, talc for dry skin, rouge, Vaseline and toilet paper for blisters, rouge and mortician's wax for ulcers (farm setting with equipment and bystanders).

INITIAL SCENE DESCRIPTION

Dispatch Information

LOCATION: Local farm
NUMBER OF VICTIMS: 1
TYPE OF SITUATION: Unknown problem
HAZARDS: None apparent
WEATHER CONDITIONS: Clear, windy day
TIME OF DAY: 1335

Scene

You are dispatched to a farm field near town. The dispatcher states that he was told only that one of the farm workers is ill. He states he has no further information because the caller spoke very "broken" English. Upon arrival, you are directed to an area next to a large storehouse. You see several people crowded around a young Latin male. He was brought from the fields by a flat car pulled by a tractor. As you and your partner collect your equipment, the foreman walks over and states, again in broken English, that his employee was splashed with a poison. He responds to your first question, "What kind of poison?", with "no comprende." A young woman who is close by begins to translate, saying that the foreman does not know the name of the poison, but he will go get the name from the 55-gallon barrel. He leaves the area and the woman begins to explain that the field crew was spraying the poison from the back of the tractor when the patient was walking next to the truck, and one of the open barrels tipped over, splashing all over him. As you arrive at the side of the patient, he is sitting up on a box near a work shed, obviously short of breath and attempting to speak to you in Spanish. The young woman says he is complaining that he cannot breathe and his mouth is burning. You observe ulcers and blisters about his lips, mouth, face, neck, and chest.

PRIMARY ASSESSMENT FINDINGS

SCENE SURVEY

- ▼ farm work area
- ▼ patient sitting up on box
- ▼ possible chemical hazard

AIRWAY/CERVICAL SPINE

- ▼ open airway
- ▼ no signs of trauma
- ▼ neck veins flat

BREATHING

- 32 breaths per minute noted, labored
- symmetrical chest rise noted
- lung sounds reveal rales, bilaterally

CIRCULATION/HEMORRHAGE CONTROL

- strong carotid pulse of 100
- no radial pulse
- capillary refill at 4 seconds
- no obvious external blood loss

DISABILITY

- (A,V,P,U) difficult to determine due to language barrier

EXPOSE AND EXAMINE

- reddish skin blisters and ulcers noted
- skin turgor poor, dry cracked skin
- skin color pale
- skin cool and dry
- weight estimated at 140 lb

SECONDARY ASSESSMENT FINDINGS

VITAL SIGNS

- respirations, 32 and labored
- pulse, 100
- blood pressure, 70/60
- ECG, a normal sinus rhythm

HISTORY

- as above, except for the following:
    - A   unable to obtain
    - M   unable to obtain
    - P   unable to obtain
    - L   unable to obtain
    - E   splashed with an unknown chemical

HEAD

- no visible trauma
- skin blisters and ulcerations of the lips and mouth

- no deformity on palpation
- pupils white and cloudy (opaque), dilated and nonreactive to light

NECK

- trachea midline
- neck veins flat
- skin ulcerations and blistering noted

CHEST

- no visible trauma
- skin ulcerations and blistering noted
- symmetrical chest wall movement
- lung sounds reveal rales, bilaterally
- no deformity, tenderness, or crepitus noted on palpation

ABDOMEN

- abdomen slightly distended
- soft, slightly tender to palpation
- (if checked, bowel sounds absent)
- pelvic rock stable

EXTREMITIES

- no deformity
- no discoloration
- no visible signs of trauma
- capillary refill delayed to 4 seconds
- no distal pulses present
- skin turgor poor, dry cracked skin
- skin color pale
- skin cool and dry to touch
- no tenderness, crepitus, or swelling
- movement of extremities equal

NEUROLOGICAL

- unable to determine accurately due to language barrier
- Glascow coma scale can not be calculated at this time:
  - eye opening, spontaneous (4)
  - verbal response, unable to obtain
  - motor response, can obtain what appears to be a normal response to verbal stimuli (6)

SENSORY EXAM

▼ no deficit in sensory or motor function

BACK

▼ no deformity
▼ no discoloration
▼ no trauma noted

Scenario Progression and Analysis: Early on in the scenario the patient begins to vomit. At some point during the course of the scenario, the foreman returns and informs the team that the chemical is paraquat. The signs and symptoms of the scenario indicate this type of poisoning. All levels of certification should be tested on the same things during this scenario. They should recognize the scene hazard and not begin treatment until the patient is decontaminated. If they fail to do so, they should become ill themselves. Once they identify the poison, they should remove any oxygen provided to the patient. If they do not know the chemistry of the agent, they should contact medical control or poison control and be advised to reduce oxygen administration. If they fail to reduce oxygen concentration, the patient's respiratory distress should increase. The patient's level of consciousness rapidly deteriorates and lapses into coma. Since this patient is also hypotensive, with lung sounds that reveal rales, the paramedics should treat this with a dopamine infusion after checking with either poison or medical control.

SUGGESTED TREATMENT

EMT-A Level:

▼ Conduct Scene Survey.
  ▼ Decontamination, as per local protocols (soap and water, diking, and so on).
▼ Conduct Primary Assessment.
▼ Airway management will probably include the application of a mask with a high administration of O_2.

THE FOREMAN RETURNS AND SAYS THE POISON IS PARAQUAT.

▼ Contact medical or poison control if unfamiliar with the poison.
▼ If high-flow O_2 has been administered, direction to remove it should be given.
▼ Conduct Secondary Assessment.

**AT THIS TIME, PATIENT VOMITS AND BECOMES
UNRESPONSIVE (WITH RESPIRATIONS STILL AT 32
AND A CAROTID PULSE OF 100 BPM).**

- ▼ Suction vigorously.
  - ▼ Hyperventilate before and after.
  - ▼ Suction only on withdrawal.
  - ▼ Suction no longer than 10 seconds.
- ▼ Airway management should include proper application of the bag-valve-mask device without O_2 administration.
  - ▼ Position patient properly.
  - ▼ Open airway with head-tilt, chin-lift method.
  - ▼ Insert naso/oropharyngeal airway.
- ▼ Reassess airway, breathing, circulation, and level of consciousness.
- ▼ Transport ASAP.
- ▼ Do not delay for ALS Unit.
- ▼ Notify appropriate receiving facility.

EMT-I Level

- ▼ Treatment is the same as above, but includes the following:
- ▼ Airway management should not include insertion of an esophageal airway.
- ▼ Establish a large-bore IV, infusing Ringer's lactate or normal saline, KVO.

EMT-P Level

- ▼ Conduct Scene Survey.
  - ▼ Decontamination, as per local protocols (soap and water, diking, and so on).
- ▼ Conduct Primary Assessment.
- ▼ Airway management will probably include the application of a mask with a high administration of O_2

**THE FOREMAN RETURNS AND SAYS
THE POISON IS PARAQUAT.**

- ▼ Contact medical or poison control if unfamiliar with the poison.
- ▼ If high-flow O_2 has been administered, direction to remove it should be given.
- ▼ Conduct Secondary Assessment.

**AT THIS TIME, PATIENT VOMITS AND BECOMES
UNRESPONSIVE (WITH RESPIRATIONS STILL AT 32
AND A CAROTID PULSE OF 100 BPM).**

- ▼ Suction vigorously.
    - ▼ Hyperventilate before and after.
    - ▼ Suction only on withdrawal.
    - ▼ Suction no longer than 10 seconds.
- ▼ Airway management should include proper application of the bag-valve-mask device without O_2 administration.
    - ▼ Position patient properly.
    - ▼ Open airway with head-tilt, chin-lift method.
    - ▼ Insert naso/oropharyngeal airway.
- ▼ Rapidly assess ECG, showing a normal sinus rhythm.
- ▼ Complete oral intubation with appropriate-sized tube.
    - ▼ No longer than 30 seconds.
    - ▼ Hyperventilate before and after.
    - ▼ Assess lung sounds.
- ▼ Reassess airway, breathing, circulation, and level of consciousness.
- ▼ Transport ASAP.
- ▼ Establish a large-bore IV, infusing Ringer's lactate or normal saline, KVO.
- ▼ Administer dopamine, as per local protocols, after contacting medical or poison control.

PATIENT'S BP = 100/70.

- ▼ Notify appropriate receiving facility.

ADDITIONAL PROBLEMS

Depending on the level of the candidate, the following problems can be added to the scenario:

1. Proper decontamination must be performed before any treatment is begun. If it is not performed, the members of the team should begin to be affected.
2. The patient could have a seizure, requiring intervention with diazepam.
3. Cardiac dysrhythmia may occur, requiring management.
4. The interpreter must leave the scene during scenario, never to return.
5. Even if the candidate does speak Spanish, it is a dialect that he or she does not understand.
6. The presenter may add any additional, underlying medical problems that he wishes to test (for example, COPD, heart disease, or hypertension).
7. The dopamine infusion could cause ectopy, requiring the proper intervention.
8. Other units may be allowed to be called in if the presenter wishes to test the effective way to manage a hazardous materials scene.
9. Any location can be given to test the candidate's street or address competency, using local running cards.

10. Any scene hazard can be incorporated at the presenter's discretion. (This is in addition to or replacement of those already mentioned.).

11. If a pulse oximeter reading is asked for by the candidate, an appropriate reading should be given.

SUMMARY

The purpose of this scenario is to identify that this patient has been exposed to a poison and that decontamination must be performed before treatment is begun. Initially, before any primary survey, a scene survey must be performed. Hazards must be identified and mitigated before the prehospital care provider rushes in to treat the patient. If not all the information is first available at the scene, then the provider should wait, or proceed with extreme caution. If the agency that provides BLS/ALS does not have the capabilities to deal with a hazard, additional resources should be summoned. You benefit the patient in no way by becoming a victim yourself.

Paraquat poisoning is rarely seen. Its toxic effects occur in the lungs, where it can cause pulmonary edema, fibrosis, and progressive respiratory failure. Unlike other poisonings, the administration of oxygen is contraindicated. The administration of supplemental oxygen will accelerate the pathophysiology of this toxic agent, and lung damage will be exacerbated. Paraquat is extremely toxic and is used as a herbicide. The management is directed at reducing the damage that the poison causes. If the provider has knowledge of this agent, he or she will not administer oxygen. But if the provider does not know about this particular poison she or he should request additional assistance in the management from medical or poison control.

Paraquat can also cause hypotension. Since the patient presented with lung sounds revealing rales, his blood pressure was treated with dopamine. Again, if the candidate is unfamiliar with any hazardous material, further assistance should be obtained.

TOXICOLOGICAL SCENARIO 2

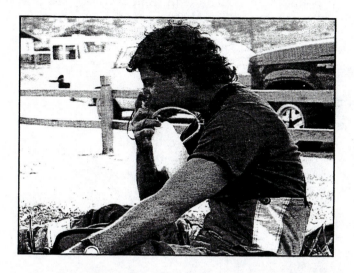

Type: Toxicological (inhalation).
Scenario moulage/prop list: Live model or mannequin, bunker gear, grease paint for flushed skin color, glycerin water for skin and hair, simple mask (fire scene with equipment and personnel).

INITIAL SCENE DESCRIPTION

Dispatch Information

LOCATION: Fire scene
NUMBER OF VICTIMS: 1
TYPE OF SITUATION: Dizziness
HAZARDS: Unknown
WEATHER CONDITIONS: Cool, clear, night
TIME OF DAY: 2334 hours

Scene

You are called to a fire scene for a firefighter who is complaining of dizziness. As you arrive, the other firefighters direct you to the patient. One explains that they "had been overhauling the building after having extinguished the fire" when the patient collapsed. This individual goes on to say that everyone removed their breathing apparatus about 2 hours before, when the smoke was still "pretty thick" and the patient had been in the structure "the whole time." You find the 35-year-old male sitting outside breathing oxygen from a simple mask. He's not sure what happened and appears confused and lethargic. His other complaints include "a pounding headache with some nausea." You attempt to walk him over to your truck, but he is unable to stand. His heavy bunker coat has been removed.

PRIMARY ASSESSMENT FINDINGS

SCENE SURVEY

- ▼ outside, fire scene
- ▼ firefighter sitting on ground breathing O_2

AIRWAY/CERVICAL SPINE

- ▼ open airway
- ▼ no signs of trauma
- ▼ neck veins slightly distended

BREATHING

- ▼ 36 breaths per minute noted, labored
- ▼ symmetrical chest rise noted
- ▼ lung sounds clear bilaterally

CIRCULATION/HEMORRHAGE CONTROL

- ▼ strong carotid pulse at 112
- ▼ strong radial pulse at 112
- ▼ capillary refill at 2 seconds
- ▼ no obvious external blood loss

DISABILITY

- ▼ (A, V, P, U) responds to verbal stimuli

EXPOSE AND EXAMINE

- ▼ no obvious deformity or discoloration
- ▼ skin turgor good
- ▼ skin color flushed
- ▼ skin hot and wet to touch
- ▼ weight estimated at 190 lb

SECONDARY ASSESSMENT FINDINGS

VITAL SIGNS

- ▼ respirations, 36 and labored
- ▼ pulse, 112 and regular

- blood pressure, 160/90
- ECG, a sinus tachycardia

HISTORY

- as above, except for the following:
    - A   none
    - M   thiazide
    - P   hypertension
    - L   normal dinner that evening
    - E   working at a fire scene without rehabilitation

HEAD

- no visible trauma
- no deformity on palpation
- pupils equal and reactive to light

NECK

- trachea midline
- neck veins slightly distended
- no deformity
- skin color flushed

CHEST

- no visible deformity
- skin flushed
- symmetrical chest wall movement
- lung sounds clear and equal bilaterally
- no deformity, tenderness, or crepitus noted on palpation

ABDOMEN

- abdomen slightly distended
- soft, slightly tender to palpation
- (if checked, bowel sounds absent)
- pelvic rock stable

EXTREMITIES

- no deformity
- no discoloration
- no visible trauma
- capillary refill at 2 seconds
- distal pulses present
- skin turgor good
- skin color flushed

- skin hot and moist to touch
- no tenderness, crepitus, or swelling
- sluggish, but movement of extremities equal

NEUROLOGICAL

- conscious, confused, becoming progressively more sluggish
- Glascow coma scale calculated at 14:
    - eye opening, spontaneous (4)
    - verbal response, confused (4)
    - motor response, obeys (6)

SENSORY EXAM

- sluggish, but no deficit in sensory or motor function

BACK

- no deformity
- no discoloration
- no trauma noted

Scenario Progression and Analysis: This patient has inhaled enough carbon monoxide to make him feel this way. Carbon monoxide poisoning is best treated by aggressive airway management and transport to a facility with a hyperbaric chamber. Midway through the scenario, the patient will have a change in his level of consciousness and become only responsive to pain. EMT-As and Is should be tested on how quickly they diagnose the problem, initiate proper airway control, and decide to transport or call for an ALS Unit. Paramedics should attempt to orally intubate this patient, unfortunately, it will be without success (due to a gag reflex). They should realize the importance of intubation in this scenario, and once they try a nasal intubation, they will be successful. If airway management is proper and complete and transport rapid, the patient should remain the same; if not, his condition should deteriorate.

SUGGESTED TREATMENT

EMT-A Level

- Conduct Scene Survey.
    - Assure that patient is far enough away from the fire scene.
    - Establish combustion source and/or combustion by-products.
- Conduct Primary Assessment

A FIREFIGHTER RETURNS AND STATES THAT ONLY PAPER AND WOOD PRODUCTS WERE ON FIRE.

- Conduct Secondary Assessment.
  - Assure that excessive clothing is removed to enhance heat loss.
- Airway management should include a change to a mask with a high administration of O_2
- Reassess airway, breathing, circulation, and level of consciousness.

**AT THIS TIME, THE PATIENT BECOMES EXTREME-
LY LETHARGIC (RESPIRATIONS REMAIN AT 36 AND
PULSE AT 112 BPM).**

- Airway management should include proper application of the bag-valve-mask device with 100% O_2 administration.
  - Position patient properly.
  - Open airway with head-tilt, chin-left method.
  - Hyperventilate patient.

**THE PATIENT WILL NOT TOLERATE
AN OROPHARYNGEAL AIRWAY DUE TO A GAG REFLEX.**

- Insert a nasopharyngeal airway.
- Reassess airway, breathing, circulation, and level of consciousness.
- Transport ASAP or call for an ALS Unit.
- Notify appropriate receiving facility.

EMT-I Level

- Treatment is the same as above, but includes the following:
- Establish a large-bore IV, infusing normal saline, as per local protocols, KVO.

EMT-P Level

- Conduct Scene Survey.
  - Assure that patient is far enough away from the fire scene.
  - Establish combustion source and/or combustion by-products.
- Conduct Primary Assessment.

**A FIREFIGHTER RETURNS AND STATES THAT ONLY
PAPER AND WOOD PRODUCTS WERE ON FIRE.**

- Conduct Secondary Assessment.
  - Assure that excessive clothing is removed to enhance heat loss.
- Airway management should include a change to a mask with a high administration of O_2

- Reassess airway, breathing, circulation, and level of consciousness.
- Assess ECG, showing a sinus tachycardia.
- Establish a large-bore IV, infusing normal saline, as per local protocols, KVO.
- Obtain glucometer/glucostrip reading (because of patient's dizziness) as per local protocols.

GLUCOSE READING = 112 MG/DL.

AT THIS TIME, THE PATIENT BECOMES EXTREMELY LETHARGIC (RESPIRATIONS REMAIN AT 36 AND PULSE AT 112 BPM).

- Airway management should include proper application of the bag-valve-mask device with 100% O_2 administration.
  - Position patient properly.
  - Open airway with head-tilt, chin-left method.
  - Insert oropharyngeal or complete oral intubation with appropriate-sized tube.

THE PATIENT WILL NOT TOLERATE ORAL INTUBATION OR ORAL AIRWAY DUE TO A GAG REFLEX.

  - Hyperventilate patient.
- Nasally intubate patient with proper technique.
  - Lubricate tube; insert in right nares.
  - Listen for air movement through the tube.
  - Assess lung sounds.
  - Continue to hyperventilate patient.
- Reassess airway, breathing, circulation, and level of consciousness.
- Transport ASAP.
- Notify appropriate receiving facility.

ADDITIONAL PROBLEMS

Depending on the level of the candidate, the following problems can be added to the scenario:
1. The patient could begin to show dysrhythmias on the monitor, requiring drug therapy.
2. The patient may lapse into coma if not rapidly diagnosed and transported.
3. The patient could vomit and aspirate, requiring vigorous suctioning.
4. The patient could develop seizure activity, requiring the proper intervention.

5. The presenter may add any additional underlying medical problems that he wishes to test (for example, COPD or heart disease).

6. The patient could also be suffering from an exposure problem, such as heat exhaustion, in combination with the carbon monoxide poisoning.

7. Any location can be given to test the candidate's street or address competency, using local running cards.

8. Any scene hazard can be incorporated at the presenter's discretion. (This is in addition to or replacement of those already mentioned.)

9. If a pulse oximeter reading is asked for by the candidate, an appropriate reading should be given.

SUMMARY

The management of this patient requires early recognition and treatment for carbon monoxide poisoning. Carbon monoxide is a colorless, odorless gas that is a by-product of the incomplete combustion of organic materials. During strenuous activity in the midst of combustion, a firefighter can develop lethal levels of carbon monoxide in his blood in less than 1 minute. The first step will be to identify the poisoning agent. Then, treatment begins with the removal of the patient from the area. After a primary survey is completed, the administration of oxygen with the highest concentration possible is indicated.

Carbon monoxide binds to hemoglobin with an affinity that is 200 to 250 times that of oxygen. Saturation of the hemoglobin molecule with carbon monoxide prevents oxygen from binding to the sites occupied by carbon monoxide. When oxygen is bound to a hemoglobin molecule that is partly saturated with carbon monoxide, it becomes bound more tightly than usual and is less likely to be released to the tissues. Tissue hypoxia results from both of these mechanisms. Additionally, at the microcellular level, carbon monoxide binds to the enzyme cytochrome oxidase, thus inhibiting the energy production necessary for all vital processes.

By increasing the oxygen content of the blood, using either 100% oxygen or hyperbaric oxygen, there will be more oxygen molecules competing for the binding sites on the hemoglobin molecule. Eventually, oxygen will replace most of the carbon monoxide molecules, allowing normal delivery of oxygen to the tissues. The most effective and quickest way to desaturate the hemoglobin is with hyperbaric oxygen; this requires that the patient be placed in a hyperbaric or decompression chamber. The increase in atmospheric pressure combined with 100% oxygen reduces the time for desaturation and excretion of carbon monoxide. Some physicians feel that even in a minor exposure patients should be placed in a hyperbaric chamber for this treatment.

Since the effects of carbon conoxide poisoning are potentially lethal in a short period of time, airway management must be aggressive. In this instance, the patient's gag reflex prevented oral intubation, so another technique, such as nasal intubation, had to be considered.

It should be noted that the cherry red color associated with carbon monoxide poisoning does not occur until saturation of hemoglobin with carbon monoxide exceeds 50%. Symptoms and signs of poisoning will occur before this level is reached.

TOXILOGICAL SCENARIO 3

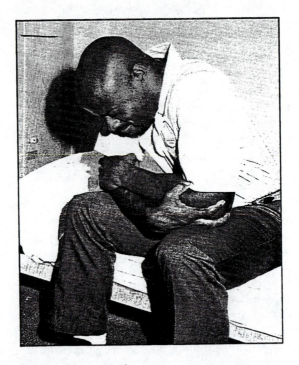

Type: Toxicological (overdose).
Scenario moulage/prop list: Live model or mannequin, apartment setting, glycerin water in spray bottle for skin (bedroom setting).

INITIAL SCENE DESCRIPTION

Dispatch Information

LOCATION: House in the suburbs
NUMBER OF VICTIMS: 1
TYPE OF SITUATION: Medical; man with joint pain
HAZARDS: None
WEATHER CONDITIONS: Clear with no traffic problems
TIME OF DAY: 2200 hours

Scene

At 2200 hours, you are dispatched to a house in the suburbs for a 22-year-old black male complaining of "severe joint pain." The pain is so intense that the patient has difficulty answering your questions. Eventually, he explains that he has a history of sickle cell anemia and denies any recent trauma. He states, "I took some pills for pain I got from a friend one hour ago." He has no idea of the type or name of the medication he took and has no pills left to show you. He insists that there is presently no way to contact the friend and that the medication has given him no relief "whatsoever." The patient's complaints and pain lead you to believe that you cannot move him at this time. His vital signs appear stable; so when you contact medical control they order 5 mg of morphine sulfate IVP and an IV of Ringer's lactate to infuse at a wide open rate. They also advise high-flow oxygen, which you had already initiated. You complete the above orders, prepare the patient for transport, and begin to move him out of the bedroom. At this time, your partner suddenly notes that the patient is no longer talking and has a respiratory rate of 5 breaths per minute.

PRIMARY ASSESSMENT FINDINGS

SCENE SURVEY

- bedroom with man on floor
- no apparent hazards

AIRWAY/CERVICAL SPINE

- airway open
- no signs of trauma
- neck veins flat

BREATHING

- 5 breaths per minute, shallow
- symmetrical chest rise
- lungs clear bilaterally, but distant

CIRCULATION/HEMORRHAGE CONTROL

- slow, weak carotid pulse at 60
- no radial pulse felt
- capillary refill delayed to 6 seconds
- no external bleeding observed

DISABILITY

- (A,V,P,U) unresponsive

EXPOSE AND EXAMINE

- ▼ no obvious deformity or discoloration
- ▼ skin turgor good
- ▼ color of mucous membranes pale
- ▼ skin cool and diaphoretic to touch
- ▼ estimated weight at 200 lb

SECONDARY ASSESSMENT FINDINGS

VITAL SIGNS

- ▼ respirations, 5 and shallow
- ▼ pulse, 60
- ▼ blood pressure, 70/50
- ▼ ECG, a normal sinus rhythm

HISTORY

- ▼ as described in the scene survey:
    - ▼ A   hydrochloride
    - ▼ M   unknown medication taken 1 hour before
    - ▼ P   sickle cell anemia and hypoglycemia "when he was a boy"
    - ▼ L   unknown
    - ▼ E O_2 initiated
    - ▼ IV Ringer's lactate started, right antecubital
    - ▼ morphine sulfate 5 mg, IVP
    - ▼ change in respiratory rate and volume
    - ▼ change in level of consciousness after medication administration

HEAD

- ▼ no visible trauma
- ▼ no deformity on palpation
- ▼ pupils constricted and nonreactive to light

NECK

- ▼ trachea midline
- ▼ neck veins flat
- ▼ no deformity
- ▼ no discoloration

CHEST

- ▼ no visible deformity
- ▼ no discoloration

- ▼ symmetrical chest wall movement
- ▼ lung sounds clear, equal bilaterally, but distant
- ▼ no deformity, tenderness, or crepitus on palpation

ABDOMEN

- ▼ abdomen nondistended
- ▼ soft, nontender to palpation
- ▼ (if checked, bowel sounds present)
- ▼ pelvic rock stable

EXTREMITIES

- ▼ no deformity
- ▼ no discoloration
- ▼ no visible signs of trauma
- ▼ capillary refill delayed to 6 seconds
- ▼ no distal pulses present
- ▼ skin turgor good
- ▼ color of mucous membranes pale
- ▼ skin cool and diaphoretic to touch
- ▼ no tenderness, crepitus, or swelling
- ▼ equal extremity movement prior to loss of consciousness

NEUROLOGICAL

- ▼ unconscious, unresponsive
- ▼ Glasgow coma scale calculated at 3:
  - ▼ eye opening, none (1)
  - ▼ verbal response, none (1)
  - ▼ motor response, none (1)

SENSORY EXAM

- ▼ unable to determine sensory or motor function

BACK

- ▼ no deformity
- ▼ no discoloration
- ▼ no trauma noted

Scenario Progression and Analysis: The patient's level of consciousness and respiratory status remain the same until naloxone is administered. Upon administration, the patient's respiratory rate increases to 10 per minute while his level of consciousness increases only slightly (moaning with painful stimuli). The patient's blood pressure should stay low throughout the treatment. Paramedics should be tested on how quickly they administer the naloxone to reverse the effects of the morphine and then readdress the airway and hypotension. If naloxone is not given or the hypotension is not addressed, then the patient should go into respiratory arrest and subsequent cardiac arrest.

SUGGESTED TREATMENT

EMT-A Level:

This scenario is directed toward EMT-paramedic level only.

EMT-I Level:

This scenario is directed toward EMT-paramedic level only.

EMT-P Level

- ▼ Conduct scene survey.
    - ▼ Search for medications.
- ▼ Conduct Primary Assessment, including rapid assessment of ECG showing a normal sinus rhythm.
- ▼ Airway management should include proper application of the bag-valve-mask device with 100% O_2 administration.
    - ▼ Position patient properly.
    - ▼ Open airway with head-tilt, chin-lift.
    - ▼ Insert naso/oropharyngeal airway.
- ▼ Administer 2 mg of naloxone IV and titrate to respiratory rate.
- ▼ Reassess ECG, airway, breathing, circulation, and level of consciousness.

AT THIS TIME, THE PATIENT'S RESPIRATIONS INCREASE TO 10 AND SHALLOW, WHILE THE PATIENT BEGINS TO RESPOND TO PAIN.

- ▼ Complete oral intubation with appropriate-sized tube.
    - ▼ Hyperventilate before and after.
    - ▼ No longer than 30 seconds.
    - ▼ Assess lung sounds.
- ▼ Conduct secondary Assessment.

AT THIS TIME, THE PATIENT'S BLOOD PRESSURE REMAINS 70/50.

- ▼ Apply pneumatic antishock garment.
- ▼ Reassess ECG, airway, breathing, circulation, and level of consciousness.

▼ Transport ASAP.

▼ Establish at least one more large-bore IV infusing Ringer's lactate, open.

▼ Draw blood sample and obtain a glucometer/glucostrip reading.

GLUCOSE READING = 100 MG/DL.

▼ Administer dopamine as per local protocols.

▼ Reassess ECG, airway, breathing, circulation, and level of consciousness.

PATIENT'S BP = 98/60.

▼ Notify appropriate receiving facility.

ADDITIONAL PROBLEMS

At the presenter's discretion, the following problems can be added to the scenario:

1. The patient can go into any cardiac dysrhythmia that you wish to test.

2. Additional difficulty of airway management can be accomplished by adding vomiting to the scenario or by having the patient unable to be intubated.

3. As a result of fluid administration, patient's airway can be compromised with pulmonary edema.

4. Make the patient's sugar reading low so that the candidate has to administer 50% dextrose.

5. After IV lines have been established, the patient can deteriorate and go into cardiac arrest to further test the candidate's knowledge.

6. Any location can be given to test the candidate's street or address competency, using local running cards.

7. Any scene hazard can be incorporated at the presenter's discretion. (This is in addition to or replacement of those already mentioned.)

8. The presenter may add any additional, underlying medical problems that he or she wishes to test (for example, COPD, heart disease, or hypertension).

SUMMARY

This patient took an excessive dose of diazepam prior to your arrival. The morphine ordered by medical control potentiated the central nervous system depression of the diazepam. Naloxone would be effective in antagonizing the effects of narcotic or synthetic narcotics drugs only. Diazepam, although a central nervous system depressant, is not a narcotic. Naloxone would not reverse diazepam's effects.

The primary complaint of the patient was joint pain caused by sickle cell anemia. The physiology of this disease causes red blood cells to change to a sickle shape due to hypoxia from any source. This cell shape clogs capillaries and blood flow through joints. The treatment is directed toward pain relief, oxygenation, and hemodilution. Pain relief is accomplished through narcotic administration. While high-flow oxygen helps reduce the sickling of red blood cells. Fluid administration will reduce the viscosity of the blood and increase perfusion.

TOXICOLOGICAL SCENARIO 4

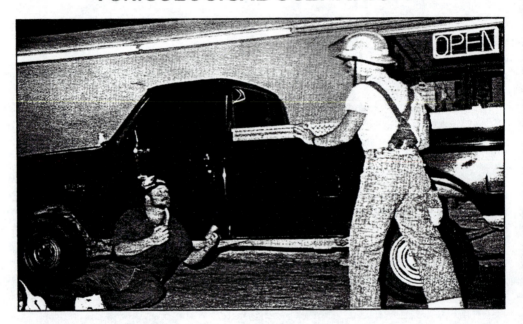

Type: Toxicological (alcohol).
Scenario moulage/prop list: Live model or mannequin, grease paint for pale skin color, glycerin water for skin, prop knife, rum or whiskey for etoh breath (parking lot setting).

INITIAL SCENE DESCRIPTION

Dispatch Information

LOCATION: Local bar parking lot
NUMBER OF VICTIMS: 1
TYPE OF SITUATION: Man acting bizarrely
HAZARDS: Unknown
WEATHER CONDITIONS: Clear, early morning
TIME OF DAY: 0211 hours

Scene

You are called to a local pub's parking lot for a man acting "bizarrely." It is just after 2:00 A.M. and you and your partners were sleeping at the time you were "beeped out". En route, you perfunctorily ask dispatch if either the police are en route or already on scene. "They are en route," the dispatcher confirms.

When you arrive you find a 45-year-old male sitting next to a parked truck. He explains that he is "not hurt," but he cannot tell you the day, month, or even what time it is. The bartender says that the man got to the bar about one hour before and only had "a couple of drinks."

The patient smells of alcohol and states, "I've had a couple of vodka tonics." And then, in the same breath, he takes out a knife and begins punching holes in the tire next to him, adding, "If you don't leave me alone I'll kill everyone, including myself."

PRIMARY ASSESSMENT FINDINGS

SCENE SURVEY

▼ parking lot
▼ man with knife, threatening harm to you and your crew andhimself

AIRWAY/CERVICAL SPINE

▼ open airway
▼ no signs of trauma
▼ neck veins flat

BREATHING

▼ 20 breaths per minute noted
▼ symmetrical chest rise noted
▼ lung sounds clear bilaterally

CIRCULATION/HEMORRHAGE CONTROL

▼ strong carotid pulse at 112
▼ strong radial pulse at 112
▼ capillary refill at 2 seconds
▼ no obvious external blood loss

DISABILITY

▼ (A, V, P, U) responsive to verbal stimuli, combative and threatening

EXPOSE AND EXAMINE

▼ no obvious deformity or discoloration
▼ skin color pale

- ▼ skin turgor good
- ▼ skin cool and diaphoretic to touch
- ▼ weight estimated at 275 lb

VITAL SIGNS

- ▼ respirations, 20
- ▼ pulse, 112
- ▼ blood pressure, 100/70
- ▼ ECG, a normal sinus rhythm

HISTORY

- ▼ as above, except for the following:
  - ▼ A unknown
  - ▼ M unknown
  - ▼ P unknown
  - ▼ L unknown
  - ▼ E drinking alcohol at a bar

HEAD

- ▼ no visible trauma
- ▼ no deformity on palpation
- ▼ pupils equal and reactive to light

NECK

- ▼ trachea midline
- ▼ neck veins flat
- ▼ no deformity
- ▼ no discoloration

CHEST

- ▼ no visible deformity
- ▼ no discoloration
- ▼ symmetrical chest wall movement
- ▼ lung sounds clear and equal bilaterally
- ▼ no deformity, tenderness, or crepitus noted on palpation

ABDOMEN

- ▼ abdomen nondistended
- ▼ soft, nontender to palpation
- ▼ (if checked, bowel sounds present)
- ▼ pelvic rock stable

EXTREMITIES

- ▾ no deformity
- ▾ no discoloration
- ▾ no visible signs of trauma
- ▾ capillary refill at 2 seconds
- ▾ strong distal pulses present
- ▾ skin turgor good
- ▾ skin color pale
- ▾ skin cool and diaphoretic to touch
- ▾ no tenderness, crepitus, or swelling
- ▾ movement of extremities equal

NEUROLOGICAL

- ▾ conscious, confused
- ▾ Glascow coma scale calculated at 14
    - ▾ eye opening, spontaneous (4)
    - ▾ verbal response, confused (4)
    - ▾ motor response, obeys (6)

SENSORY EXAM

- ▾ no deficit in sensory or motor function

BACK

- ▾ no deformity
- ▾ no discoloration
- ▾ no trauma noted

Scenario Progression and Analysis: This is a patient who has been become both violent and suicidal. The key factor here is that all prehospital care providers should wait for the police to arrive and then examine the patient after he has been subdued and restrained. This patient is not a psychiatric patient, but a noninsulin-dependent diabetic who is suffering from hypoglycemia. EMT-As and Is should be tested on their scene survey, concern for safety, rapid diagnosis, administration of glucogel (as per local protocols), and the decision to transport or call for an ALS Unit. Paramedics, with their glucometers, will have a diagnostic edge on those without, but diagnosis and basic treatment (50% dextrose, IV, for the medics, in this case) should be the same.

SUGGESTED TREATMENT

EMT-A Level

- ▾ Conduct Scene Survey.
    - ▾ Keep distance.

- ▼ Call for the police department and await their arrival.
- ▼ Help the police restrain the patient as per local protocols.
- ▼ Conduct Primary Assessment.
- ▼ Conduct Secondary Assessment.
- ▼ Airway management should include the administration of O_2 via a nasal canula.
- ▼ Reassess airway, breathing, circulation, and level of consciousness.
- ▼ Administer glucogel, as per local protocols.
- ▼ Reassess airway, breathing, circulation, and level of consciousness.
- ▼ Transport or call for an ALS Unit.
- ▼ Notify appropriate receiving facility.
- ▼ Monitor patient's level of consciousness.

AT THIS TIME, THE PATIENT BECOMES LESS VIOLENT AND BEGINS TO TALK MORE RATIONALLY, SAYING THAT HE IS A NONINSULIN-DEPENDENT DIABETIC TAKING CHLORPROPAMIDE.

EMT-I Level

- ▼ Treatment is the same as above, but includes the following:
- ▼ Establish a large-bore IV, infusing dextrose 5%, KVO.

EMT-P Level

- ▼ Conduct Scene Survey.
    - ▼ Keep distance.
    - ▼ Call for the police department and await their arrival.
    - ▼ Help the police restrain the patient as per local protocols.
- ▼ Conduct Primary Assessment.
- ▼ Conduct Secondary Assessment.
- ▼ Airway management should include the administration of O_2 via a nasal canula.
- ▼ Reassess airway, breathing, circulation, and level of consciousness.
- ▼ Draw blood and obtain glucometer/glucostrip reading.
- ▼ Establish a large-bore IV, infusing 5% dextrose, KVO.

GLUCOSE READING = 42 MG/DL.

- ▼ Administer dextrose 50%, IV.
- ▼ Reassess airway, breathing, circulation, and level of consciousness.

AT THIS TIME, THE PATIENT BECOMES LESS VIOLENT AND BEGINS TO TALK MORE RATIONALLY SAYING THAT HE IS A NONINSULIN-DEPENDENT DIABETIC TAKING CHLORPROPAMIDE.

▼ Transport.
▼ Notify appropriate receiving facility.
▼ Monitor patient's level of consciousness.

ADDITIONAL PROBLEMS

Depending on the level of the candidate, the following problems can be added to the scenario:

1. The patient could have a seizure or become unresponsive, due to his hypoglycemia, sometime during the scenario.
2. The patient may lapse back into a violent, confused state, requiring the candidate to obtain another glucose reading and give another ampule of dextrose 50%.
3. The secondary survey may reveal some signs of trauma, requiring the candidate to cervically immobilize the patient, as well as possibly changing the restraining technique used if it interferes with the immobilization. (This may include signs of a head injury, and seizures can follow.)
4. This patient could also exhibit some signs of a CVA.
5. Any additional medical complaint can follow once the patient has become more coherent (for example, chest pain).
6. Any location can be given to test the candidate's street or address competency, using local running cards.
7. Any scene hazard can be incorporated at the presenter's discretion. (This is in addition to or replacement of those already mentioned.)

SUMMARY

This scenario presents the provider with the possibility of personal injury if a scene survey is not done correctly. This situation requires the candidate to recognize that this patient is both verbally abusive and potentially violent and, if carried further, the scene could escalate to physical violence and harm to the providers. The candidate should secure adequate assistance from whatever sources are available before beginning any treatment of this patient. The scenario also emphasizes the need to fully evaluate the patient and not just assume that he is "crazy." This patient's aggressive behavior is caused by hypoglycemia and alcohol use. If the patient is simply restrained and not evaluated, then the cause of the behavior could be missed. Hypoglycemia will cause brain damage if left untreated.

Chapter 6

TRAUMA SCENARIOS

TRAUMA SCENARIO 1

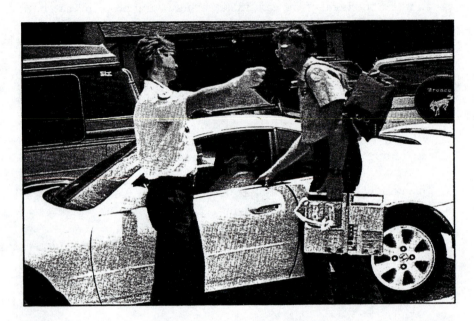

Type: Trauma.
Scenario moulage/prop list: Live model or mannequin, live model for other paramedic role, cervical collar (motor vehicle setting).

INITIAL SCENE DESCRIPTION

Dispatch Information

LOCATION: Residential street

NUMBER OF VICTIMS: 2

TYPE OF SITUATION: Car versus car, one unit on scene already

HAZARDS: Unknown

WEATHER CONDITIONS: Cool, rainy evening

TIME OF DAY: 1903 hours

Scene

You are called to the scene of an auto accident by another unit. Upon arrival, the head paramedic of the other unit directs you to a compact car with moderate damage to the front-passenger side door. He explains that the 35-year-old male driver is your patient, because they have one of a more critical nature in the other car. He quickly gives you the patient "run down." "This patient is basic life support, all the way," he says. "Pulse is 72, blood pressure is 130/80...seems real stable...we just haven't done a complete secondary survey on him yet." You see the patient sitting in the driver's seat with a cervical collar already applied.

PRIMARY ASSESSMENT FINDINGS

SCENE SURVEY

▼ residential street
▼ man sitting in driver's seat with seatbelt on and cervical collar applied
▼ no apparent hazards

AIRWAY/CERVICAL SPINE

▼ open airway
▼ no signs of trauma
▼ neck veins flat

BREATHING

▼ 20 breaths per minute noted
▼ symmetrical chest rise noted
▼ lungs clear bilaterally

CIRCULATION/HEMORRHAGE CONTROL

▼ strong carotid pulse of 68
▼ strong radial pulse of 68
▼ capillary refill at 2 seconds
▼ no obvious external blood loss

DISABILITY

▼ (A, V, P, U) alert

EXPOSE AND EXAMINE

▼ no obvious deformity or discoloration
▼ skin turgor good
▼ skin color normal

- skin warm and dry to touch
- weight estimated at 160 lb

SECONDARY ASSESSMENT FINDINGS

VITAL SIGNS

- respirations, 20
- pulse, 68
- blood pressure, 130/70
- ECG, a normal sinus rhythm

HISTORY

- as above, except for the following:
    - A   methiolate
    - M   none
    - P   foot surgery
    - L   lunch at noon
    - E   T-bone auto accident with moderate damage

HEAD

- no visble trauma
- no deformity on palpation
- no CSF noted
- no Battle's Signs or raccoon's eyes
- pupils equal and reactive to light

NECK

- trachea midline
- neck veins flat
- no deformity
- no discoloration

CHEST

- no deformity
- no discoloration
- symmetrical chest wall movement
- lung sounds clear and equal bilaterally
- no deformity, tenderness, or crepitus noted on palpation

ABDOMEN

- abdomen nondistended
- soft, nontender to palpation

▼ (if checked, bowel sounds present)
▼ pelvic rock stable

EXTREMITIES

▼ no deformity
▼ no discoloration
▼ no visible signs of trauma
▼ capillary refill at 2 seconds
▼ strong distal pulses present
▼ skin turgor good
▼ skin color normal
▼ skin warm and dry to touch
▼ no tenderness, crepitus, or swelling
▼ movement of upper extremities limited to shoulders and biceps with a weak hand grip
▼ no sensation or movement noted in lower extremities

NEUROLOGICAL

▼ conscious, alert
▼ Glascow coma scale calculated at 15:
   ▼ eye opening, spontaneous (4)
   ▼ verbal response, oriented (5)
   ▼ motor response, obeys (6)

SENSORY EXAM

▼ no motor function of lower extremities, with limited function of upper extremities
▼ loss of sensation below the elbows and below the upper chest

BACK

▼ no deformity
▼ no discoloration
▼ no trauma noted

Scenario Progression and Analysis: The candidate should complete a Secondary Assessment to find that this patient has no movement and loss of sensation of his lower extremities. The patient should complain of this only after the assessment has begun. All EMTs should properly immobilize this patient and take precautions in moving him. If this is not done, the patient's loss of motor function should worsen. If BTLS/PHTLS guidelines are followed, the patient's condition should remain the same.

SUGGESTED TREATMENT

EMT-A Level

- ▼ Conduct Scene Survey.
- ▼ Conduct Primary Assessment.
- ▼ Maintain cervical spine with manual immobilization.
- ▼ Conduct Secondary Assessment.
- ▼ Apply extrication device.
- ▼ Apply cervical immobilization devices and gingerly extricate patient, placing him on a long backboard.
- ▼ Reassess airway, breathing, circulation, level of consciousness, and neurological status.
- ▼ Administer oxygen, as per local protocols.
- ▼ Transport or call for an ALS Unit.
- ▼ Notify appropriate receiving facility.
- ▼ Monitor neurological status.

EMT-I Level

- ▼ Treatment is the same as above, but includes the following:
- ▼ Establish a large-bore IV, as per local protocols.

EMT-P Level

- ▼ Conduct Scene Survey.
- ▼ Conduct Primary Assessment.
- ▼ Maintain cervical spine with manual immobilization.
- ▼ Conduct Secondary Assessment.
- ▼ Apply extrication device.
- ▼ Apply cervical immobilization devices and gingerly extricate patient, placing him on a long backboard.
- ▼ Reassess airway, breathing, circulation, level of consciousness, and neurological status.
- ▼ Administer oxygen, as per local protocols.
- ▼ Establish a large-bore IV, as per local protocols.
- ▼ Assess ECG.
- ▼ Transport.
- ▼ Notify appropriate receiving facility.
- ▼ Monitor neurological status.

ADDITIONAL PROBLEMS

Depending on the level of the candidate, the following problems can be added to the scenario:

1. The patient could have any variety of Secondary Assessment problems.

2. Any history (such as diabetes) can be given initially, but the proper treatment for the history should be followed during the management (that is, blood drawn, 50% dextrose given).

3. Any location can be given to test the candidate's street or address competency, using local running cards.

4. Any scene hazard can be incorporated at the presenter's discretion. (This is in addition to or replacement of those already mentioned.)

SUMMARY

In this scenario the candidates should start with a primary survey, even though they have been told that a primary survey has been done. The primary survey confirms the findings of the previous assessment, but the management that is initiated in this primary survey is a most important point. The initial management is airway and cervical spine immobilization. If the candidate takes for granted that he does not need to perform a primary survey, he may very well miss this early intervention. If the cervical spine is not immobilized manually in addition to the cervical collar, further injury of the cord could occur. *No single immobilization device by itself is sufficient.* True immobilization requires a cervical collar and some other device in combination. The candidate should recognize that the collar is not able to truly immobilize the cervical spine and should begin manual stabilization from the beginning. Once the Primary Assessment is completed, the Secondary Assessment could begin in the vehicle, or the candidate may choose a rapid extrication if he finds the loss of motor function. The removal of the patient can be with or without extrication devices, depending on local protocols. But if the candidate elects to perform a rapid extrication without a device, then meticulous manual stabilization of the cervical spine must be maintained during this procedure.

Once the Secondary Assessment has begun, the candidate should continue cervical spine immobilization. Depending on local trauma protocols, the severity or priority of the patient should be upgraded once the loss of motor function is identified. If the candidate does not recognize the loss of motor function until the Secondary Assessment, he should upgrade the patient priority and begin preparation for transport (load and go). The Secondary Assessment should be completed en route to the hospital in this case.

This patient is suffering from a C5-C6 fracture, which is one of the most common sites of injury in trauma patients.

TRAUMA SCENARIO 2

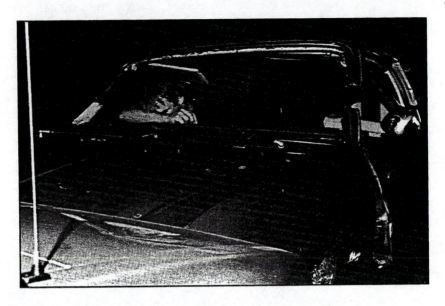

Type: Trauma with multiple patients (motor vehicle and highway setting).
Scenario moulage/prop list: Three live models or mannequins:
Patient 1, grease paint for contusion around temple area
Patient 2, mortician's wax for large laceration on forehead, raw corn (broken teeth) and red food coloring (blood) in mouth, grease paint for pale skin color and fracture of right humerus with angulation, grease paint contusion (trachea), glycerin water for skin.
Patient 3, mortician's wax for numerous lacerations to face and arms, grease paint for pale skin color and deformity right rib area, glycerin water in spray bottle for skin.

INITIAL SCENE DESCRIPTION

Dispatch Information

LOCATION: N/A
NUMBER OF VICTIMS: N/A
TYPE OF SITUATION: N/A
HAZARDS: N/A
WEATHER CONDITIONS: Rainy, early morning
TIME OF DAY: 0303 hours

Scene

It's about 3:00 A.M. and you are returning from a local hospital after transporting a woman with "chest pains." You get off the interstate, proceeding cautiously, since it has just rained and the roads are ominously slick. Your partners notice that two cars have been involved in an accident up the road, obviously just a minute or two prior to your arrival. You notify dispatch. Your unit is parked so as to block any oncoming traffic. After getting your equipment, you hustle over to the cars that have seemingly hit head on. Car A has relatively minor damage, while car B has massive damage. There are 3 patients altogether. The driver (patient 1) of car A is already out of his vehicle walking around, complaining of neck pain. There are no other passengers in car A. One of your partners yells over from car B, saying that he has two patients in that vehicle, "one unconscious with difficulty breathing " (patient 2) "and one who is apneic and pulseless" (patient 3). You hurriedly contact the dispatcher and she advises that no other units are able to respond for assistance.

PRIMARY ASSESSMENT FINDINGS: PATIENT 1, A 30-YEAR-OLD MALE

SCENE SURVEY

- major road
- patient walking around
- possible traffic hazard

AIRWAY/CERVICAL SPINE

- open airway
- neck veins slightly distended
- signs of trauma

BREATHING

- 20 breaths per minute noted
- symmetrical chest rise noted
- lung sounds clear bilaterally

CIRCULATION/HEMORRHAGE CONTROL

- rapid carotid pulse at 104
- rapid radial pulse at 104
- capillary refill at 2 seconds
- no obvious external blood loss

DISABILITY

- (A, V, P, U) alert

EXPOSE AND EXAMINE

- small contusion noted to left temple
- skin turgor good

- ▼ skin color normal
- ▼ skin warm and dry to touch
- ▼ weight estimated at 160 lb

SECONDARY ASSESSMENT FINDINGS: PATIENT 1

VITAL SIGNS

- ▼ respirations, 20
- ▼ pulse, 104
- ▼ blood pressure, 120/60
- ▼ ECG, a sinus tachycardia

HISTORY

- ▼ as above, except for the following:
  - ▼ A unknown
  - ▼ M unknown
  - ▼ P unknown
  - ▼ L unknown
  - ▼ E auto accident

HEAD

- ▼ contusion to left temple
- ▼ no deformity on palpation
- ▼ no Battle's signs, raccoon's eyes, or CSF noted
- ▼ pupils equal and reactive to light

NECK

- ▼ trachea midline
- ▼ neck veins slightly distended
- ▼ no deformity
- ▼ no discoloration

CHEST

- ▼ no deformity
- ▼ no discoloration
- ▼ symmetrical chest wall movement
- ▼ lung sounds clear and equal bilaterally
- ▼ no crepitus or tenderness on palpation

ABDOMEN

- ▼ abdomen nondistended
- ▼ soft, nontender to palpation

- ▾ (if checked, bowel sounds present)
- ▾ pelvic rock stable

EXTREMITIES

- ▾ no deformity
- ▾ no discoloration
- ▾ no visible signs of trauma
- ▾ capillary refill at 2 seconds
- ▾ distal pulses present
- ▾ skin turgor good
- ▾ skin color normal
- ▾ skin warm and dry to touch
- ▾ no tenderness, crepitus, or swelling
- ▾ movement of extremities equal

NEUROLOGICAL

- ▾ conscious, alert
- ▾ Glascow coma scale calculated at 15:
  - ▾ eye opening, spontaneous (4)
  - ▾ verbal response, oriented, (5)
  - ▾ motor response, obeys (6)

SENSORY EXAM

- ▾ no deficit in sensory or motor function

BACK

- ▾ no deformity
- ▾ no discoloration
- ▾ no trauma noted

PRIMARY ASSESSMENT FINDINGS: PATIENT 2, 25-YEAR-OLD-MALE

SCENE SURVEY

- ▾ major road
- ▾ sitting in driver's seat
- ▾ possible traffic hazard
- ▾ fluids leaking from vehicle

AIRWAY/CERVICAL SPINE

- ▾ partially obstructed airway
- ▾ disruption of front teeth with bleeding noted in mouth

- contusion of upper neck
- bruising and swelling noted above Adam's apple
- neck veins flat

BREATHING

- 44 breaths per minute noted, labored
- symmetrical chest rise noted
- lung sounds clear bilaterally

CIRCULATION/HEMORRHAGE CONTROL

- rapid carotid pulse at 132
- no radial pulse
- capillary refill delayed to 4 seconds
- some obvious external blood loss from laceration of forehead and from mouth

DISABILITY

- (A, V, P, U) responsive only to pain

EXPOSE AND EXAMINE

- large laceration of forehead
- skin turgor good
- skin color pale
- skin cool and diaphoretic to touch
- weight estimated at 200 lb

SECONDARY ASSESSMENT FINDINGS: PATIENT 2

VITAL SIGNS

- respirations, 44, obviously labored
- pulse, 132
- blood pressure, 60/p
- ECG, a sinus tachycardia

HISTORY

- as above, except for the following:
    - A   unknown
    - M   unknown
    - P   unknown

- ▼ L unknown
- ▼ E auto accident

HEAD

- ▼ large laceration of forehead
- ▼ no deformity on palpation
- ▼ disruption of front teeth
- ▼ some bleeding noted from mouth
- ▼ no Battle's signs, raccoon's eyes, or CSF noted
- ▼ pupils equal and reactive to light

NECK

- ▼ trachea midline
- ▼ neck veins flat
- ▼ bruising and swelling noted above Adam's apple

CHEST

- ▼ no visible deformity
- ▼ no discoloration
- ▼ symmetrical chest wall movement
- ▼ lung sounds clear and equal bilaterally
- ▼ no deformity, crepitus, or tenderness on palpation

ABDOMEN

- ▼ abdomen distended
- ▼ rigid, nontender to palpation
- ▼ (if checked, bowel sounds absent)
- ▼ pelvic rock stable

EXTREMITIES

- ▼ severe angulation of right humerus
- ▼ closed swelling with crepitus in same area
- ▼ no deformity noted to others
- ▼ no discoloration noted to other extremities
- ▼ capillary refill delayed to 4 seconds
- ▼ no distal pulses present
- ▼ skin turgor good
- ▼ skin color pale
- ▼ skin cool and diaphoretic to touch
- ▼ movement of extremities equal

NEUROLOGICAL

▼ stuporous, responsive only to painful stimuli
▼ Glascow coma scale calculated at 6:
  ▼ eye opening, none (1)
  ▼ verbal response, none (1)
  ▼ motor response, withdraws (4)

SENSORY EXAM

▼ withdrawal from painful stimuli and moves all extremities

BACK

▼ no deformity
▼ no discoloration
▼ no trauma noted

PRIMARY ASSESSMENT FINDINGS: PATIENT 3, A 50-YEAR-OLD MALE

SCENE SURVEY

▼ major road
▼ sitting in passenger's seat
▼ possible traffic hazard
▼ fluids leaking from vehicle

AIRWAY/CERVICAL SPINE

▼ no breathing
▼ multiple lacerations about face and arms
▼ neck veins flat

BREATHING

▼ no breathing
▼ no chest rise

CIRCULATION/HEMMORAGE

▼ no carotid pulse
▼ no radial pulse
▼ capillary refill immeasurable
▼ no active bleeding

DISABILITY

▼ (A, V, P, U) unresponsive

EXPOSE AND EXAMINE

▼ many lacerations to face and arms
▼ skin color extremely pale

- ▼ skin turgor good
- ▼ skin cool and diaphoretic to touch
- ▼ weight estimated at 155 lb

SECONDARY ASSESSMENT FINDINGS: PATIENT 3

VITAL SIGNS

- ▼ respirations, 0
- ▼ pulse, 0
- ▼ blood pressure, 0
- ▼ ECG, asystole

HISTORY

- ▼ as above, except for the following:
  - ▼ A unknown
  - ▼ M unknown
  - ▼ P unknown
  - ▼ L unknown
  - ▼ E auto accident

HEAD

- ▼ lacerations to face
- ▼ crepitus on palpation of frontal portion of skull
- ▼ Battle's signs noted
- ▼ no raccoon's eyes or CSF noted
- ▼ pupils unequal and nonreactive to light

NECK

- ▼ trachea midline
- ▼ neck veins flat
- ▼ no deformity
- ▼ no discoloration

CHEST

- ▼ no deformity
- ▼ no discoloration
- ▼ no chest wall movement
- ▼ lung sounds absent
- ▼ crepitus on palpation left rib area with several fractures noted

ABDOMEN

- ▼ abdomen distended
- ▼ rigid, nontender to palpation

▾ (if checked, bowel sounds absent)
▾ pelvic rock unstable

EXTREMITIES

▾ no deformity
▾ no discoloration
▾ capillary refill is immeasurable
▾ no distal pulses present
▾ skin turgor good
▾ skin color extremely pale
▾ skin cool and diaphoretic to touch
▾ no tenderness, crepitus, or swelling to others
▾ no movement of extremities

NEUROLOGICAL

▾ unconscious, unresponsive
▾ Glascow coma scale calculated at 3:
    ▾ eye opening, spontaneous (1)
    ▾ verbal response, oriented (1)
    ▾ motor response, obeys (1)

SENSORY EXAM

▾ unable to determine sensory or motor function

BACK

▾ no deformity
▾ no discoloration
▾ no trauma noted

Scenario Progression and Analysis: Since there is only one unit, the key here is to immediately pronounce patient 3 "Dead on Scene." Patient 1 is extremely stable and patient 2 is extremely unstable. EMT-As and Is should be tested on proper triage and adequate organization in treating the other two patients. Patient 1 should be evaluated, spinally immobilized, and then moved alongside of patient 2. Spinal immobilization and rapid extrication should be the initial treatment for patient 2 (since he is suffering from hypovolemia due to hemorrhagic shock). Subsequent treatment should include ventilation with 100% O$_2$ and antishock garment application. The decision to transport is of utmost importance since patient 2 has a crushed larynx and the airway cannot be truly stabilized by EMT-As and Is. For the paramedics, patient 2's breathing should deteriorate until either a cricothyrotomy or a transtracheal jet insufflation is performed. If BTLS/PHTLS guidelines are followed, the patients should remain the same. If not, either viable patient can deteriorate in accordance with their injuries.

SUGGESTED TREATMENTFOR PATIENT 1

EMT-A Level

- ▼ Conduct Scene Survey.
  - ▼ Contact dispatch to expedite police response.
- ▼ Conduct Primary Assessment.
- ▼ Maintain cervical spine with manual immobilization.
- ▼ Apply cervical immobilization devices and secure patient to backboard.
- ▼ Move patient near patient 2.
- ▼ Consider oxygen therapy via nasal canula.
- ▼ Conduct Secondary Assessment.

EMT-I Level

- ▼ Treatment is the same as above.

EMT-P Level

- ▼ Conduct Scene Survey.
  - ▼ Contact dispatch to expedite police response.
- ▼ Conduct Primary Assessment.
- ▼ Maintain cervical spine with manual immobilization.
- ▼ Apply cervical immobilization devices and secure patient to backboard.
- ▼ Move patient near patient 2.
- ▼ Consider oxygen therapy via nasal canula.
- ▼ Conduct Secondary Assessment.

SUGGESTED TREATMENT FOR PATIENT 2

EMT-A Level

- ▼ Conduct Scene Survey.
  - ▼ Contact dispatch to expedite police response.
  - ▼ Identify vehicle fluids as a hazard and locate a treatment area at a safe distance.
- ▼ Conduct Primary Assessment.
  - ▼ Stop any active bleeding.
- ▼ Suction vigorously.
  - ▼ Hyperventilate before and after.
  - ▼ Suction only on withdrawal.
  - ▼ Suction no longer than 10 seconds.
- ▼ Airway management should include proper application of the bag-valve-mask device with 100% O_2 administration.

- ▼ Position patient properly.
- ▼ Open airway with modified jaw thrust method.
- ▼ Insert oropharyngeal airway.
- ▼ Hyperventilate patient.
- ▼ Maintain cervical spine manually during and after airway management.
- ▼ Secure patient with cervical immobilization devices to backboard.
- ▼ Conduct MAST survey and apply pneumatic antishock garment as per local protocols.
- ▼ Reassess airway, breathing, circulation, and level of consciousness.
- ▼ Transport ASAP or call for an ALS Unit.
- ▼ Notify appropriate receiving facility.
- ▼ Conduct Secondary Assessment.

EMT-I Level

- ▼ Treatment is the same as above, but includes the following:
- ▼ Apply automatic external defibrillator, as per local protocols.
- ▼ Establish at least two large-bore IVs of normal saline or Ringer's lactate, open.
- ▼ Reassess airway, breathing, circulation, and level of consciousness.
- ▼ esophageal airway should *not* be used due to upper airway bleeding.

EMT-P Level

- ▼ Conduct Scene Survey.
    - ▼ Contact dispatch to expedite police response.
    - ▼ Identify vehicle fluids as a hazard and locate a treatment area at a safe distance.
- ▼ Conduct Primary Assessment, including a rapid assessment of ECG, showing a sinus tachycardia.
    - ▼ Stop any active bleeding.
- ▼ Suction vigorously.
    - ▼ Hyperventilate before and after.
    - ▼ Suction only on withdrawal.
    - ▼ Suction no longer than 10 seconds.
- ▼ Airway management should include proper application of the bag-valve-mask device with 100% O_2 administration.
    - ▼ Position patient properly.
    - ▼ Open airway with modified jaw thrust method.
    - ▼ Insert oropharyngeal airway.
    - ▼ Hyperventilate patient.
- ▼ Maintain cervical spine manually during and after airway management.
- ▼ Complete oral intubation with appropriate-sized tube.

UNABLE TO INTUBATE PATIENT DUE TO AIRWAY OBSTRUCTION FROM CRUSHED LARYNX. UNABLE EVEN TO VISUALIZE CORDS. PATIENT'S RESPIRATIONS ARE NOW 12/MINUTE.

- ▼ Perform cricothyrotomy or transtracheal jet insufflation, as per local protocols.
- ▼ Reassess ECG, airway, breathing, circulation, and level of consciousness.
- ▼ Secure patient with cervical immobilization devices to backboard.
- ▼ Conduct MAST survey and apply pneumatic antishock garment.
- ▼ Reassess ECG, airway, breathing, circulation, and level of consciousness.
- ▼ Transport ASAP.
- ▼ Establish at least two large-bore IVs of normal saline or Ringer's lactate, open.
- ▼ Reassess ECG, airway, breathing, circulation, and level of consciousness.
- ▼ Notify appropriate receiving facility.
- ▼ Conduct Secondary Assessment.

SUGGESTED TREATMENT FOR PATIENT 3

EMT-A Level

- ▼ Conduct Scene Survey.
  - ▼ Contact dispatch to expedite police response.
- ▼ Conduct Primary Assessment
- ▼ Decision not to resuscitate patient, following local triage guidelines.
- ▼ Cover patient
  - ▼ Apply triage tag, if possible.

EMT-I Level

- ▼ Actions are the same as above.

EMT-P Level

- ▼ Conduct Scene Survey.
  - ▼ Contact dispatch to expedite police response.
- ▼ Conduct Primary Assessment.
- ▼ Decision not to resuscitate patient, following local triage guidelines.
- ▼ Cover patient
  - ▼ Apply triage tag, if possible.

ADDITIONAL PROBLEMS

Depending on the level of the candidate, the following problems can be added to the scenario:

1. Absent lungs sounds with hyperresonance on one chest side can be given as a sign of patient 2, requiring the candidate to perform a decompression of the chest, as well as a cricothyrotomy.
2. The cricothyrotomy/transtracheal jet insufflation can be made to be difficult so that the candidate must make the decision whether to stay on scene or go
3. Any history (such as diabetes) can be given for patient 1, but the proper treatment for the history should be followed during the management (that is, blood drawn, 50% dextrose given).
4. Patient 2 could eventually go into cardiac arrest.
5. Patient 2 could have the signs of a head injury, as well, and seizures may follow.
6. Patient 1 could have more serious, hidden injuries.
7. Another unit could respond to test other individuals.
8. Any location can be given to test the candidate's street or address competency, using local running cards.
9. Any scene hazard can be incorporated at the presenter's discretion. (This is in addition to or replacement of those already mentioned.)
10. Patients 2 and 3 could need to be extricated.
11. If a pulse oximeter reading is asked for by the candidate, an appropriate reading should be given.

SUMMARY

Most prehospital care providers have been taught the concepts of major incident command. Some agencies may even practice the system as it relates to EMS. The most common types of major incidents that are practiced involve natural or man-made disasters of a large scale (airliner crash, tornados, earthquakes, floods, fires, hazardous materials, incidents, and hurricanes). Fortunately, these types of major incidents are rare. There are several major incidents that are frequently seen, but seldom practiced, since they occur on a much smaller scale. Yet, these can tax a system's equipment and personnel (for example, multiple-vehicle accidents, drive-by shootings, and bus accidents). In most cases, the number of patients is fewer than 10, although any number of patients can be overwhelming if the system is small and additional resources are limited or geographically distant.

Even if a system practices this type of drill frequently, it is often difficult for most providers to recognize the smaller major incident. The provider must switch priorities in the major incident. This change must be recognized and initiated during this scenario. In most cases that are not major incidents, the provider will attempt to resuscitate a patient who is in cardiac arrest or near cardiac arrest and exhaust all available treatment. But during a major incident, even at the smaller scale, the provider must change the priorities of her or his treatment. The patient that would normally require all the paramedic's efforts and resources to resuscitate will need to be tagged and given the lowest priority for treatment in the major incident. This is often difficult for the providers to do. They are comfortable with resuscitation and treatment of the dead or near dead and tend to go to the worst patient and begin resuscitation in any incident. The process of triage should be discussed and the concept of incident command reviewed if the candidates tested on this scenario treats the dying patient. The goal of this scenario is to recognize that this is a small-scale major incident and to begin to triage the patients. The two viable patients should be recognized and treatment begun on each. The dying patient should be triaged and tagged as the last patient for treatment and transport.

To summarize, the provider should first recognize that this scene is a major incident, initiate Incident Command System, call for assistance, and begin by triaging the patients with priority for treatment and transport. When triaging, they should perform only a Primary Assessment on each patient and then bring both viable patients to a single treatment area. Rapid stabilization and transport can then be accomplished.

TRAUMA SCENARIO 3

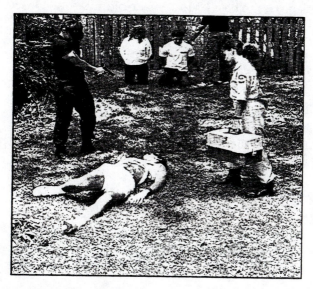

Type: Combination—trauam, medical.
Scenario moulage/prop list: Live model or mannequin, live model for police role, grease paint for pale skin color, glycerin water for skin, burned clothes, toilet paper, Vaseline and cigarette ashes for burns, rouge for frature, felt-tip marker for needle tracks (residential setting).

INITIAL SCENE DESCRIPTION

Dispatch Information

LOCATION: Single-family residence in the inner city
NUMBER OF VICTIMS: 1
TYPE OF SITUATION: Burn patient
HAZARDS: Possible fire
WEATHER CONDITIONS: Overcast, cool
TIME OF DAY: 1600 hours

Scene

You are dispatched to a single-family residence in the inner city for a burn patient. There are multiple police units on scene. Additional information is given to you, as you arrive, that the patient has been removed from "the structure on fire." Once you get out of your vehicle with your equipment, you are directed to the treatment area by the SWAT incident commander, who explains that they were on a routine "raid of a drug house." When the SWAT team arrived, they attempted to enter the house unannounced, but found they had no reasonable access, so they proceeded with some diversionary tactics to "gain forcible entry," including the use of "flashbangs," which possibly started the fire and possibly resulted in a subsequent explosion. It takes you almost 3 minutes to reach the patient, who appears to be a 25-to 30 year-old male, unconscious, lying supine in a safe area. His clothes are still smoldering.

PRIMARY ASSESSMENT FINDINGS

SCENE SURVEY

- ▼ scene appears safe
- ▼ large crowd of police
- ▼ man supine on ground along with other suspects with no injuries

AIRWAY/CERVICAL SPINE

- ▼ airway open
- ▼ singed nose hair
- ▼ burns around mouth
- ▼ neck veins flat

BREATHING

- ▼ 8 breaths per minute, shallow
- ▼ symmetrical chest rise
- ▼ bilateral wheezing

CIRCULATION/HEMORRHAGE CONTROL

- rapid, weak carotid pulse at 120
- rapid, weak radial pulse at 120
- capillary refill delayed to 4 seconds
- no obvious external blood loss

DISABILITY

- (A, V, P, U) unconscious, responds to painful stimuli

EXPOSE AND EXAMINE

- skin color pale
- skin turgor poor
- skin cool and diaphoretic to touch
- second- and third-degree burns to chest and arms
- weight estimated at 190 lb

SECONDARY ASSESSMENT FINDINGS

VITAL SIGNS

- respirations, 8
- pulse, 120
- blood pressure, 90 by palpation
- ECG, a sinus tachycardia

HISTORY

- as above, except for the following:
    - A   unknown
    - M   unknown
    - P   possible drug user
    - L   unknown
    - E   fire and explosion

HEAD

- singed nose hairs and burns around mouth
- no deformity on palpation
- no Battle's signs, raccoon's eyes, or CSF noted
- pupils pinpoint

NECK

- trachea midline
- neck veins flat

- ▼ no deformity
- ▼ no discoloration

CHEST

- ▼ second- and third-degree burns involving both pectoral muscles, estimated at 9%
- ▼ symmetrical chest wall movement
- ▼ lung sounds reveal wheezing bilaterally
- ▼ no deformity, tenderness, or crepitus on palpation

ABDOMEN

- ▼ abdomen nondistended
- ▼ soft, nontender to palpation
- ▼ (if checked, bowel sounds present)
- ▼ pelvic rock with crepitus noted

EXTREMITIES

- ▼ left leg angulated at femur area with pulses and sensation present, distally, but limited range of motion noted
- ▼ crepitus noted to left femur area
- ▼ second- and third-degree burns involving both arms, totally (18%)
- ▼ no trauma to right leg
- ▼ numerous needle tracks noted on legs
- ▼ capillary refill at 4 seconds
- ▼ weak, distal pulses present
- ▼ skin turgor poor
- ▼ skin color pale
- ▼ skin cool and diaphoretic to touch
- ▼ no tenderness, crepitus, or swelling to other extremities
- ▼ movement of all other extremities equal

NEUROLOGICAL

- ▼ unconscious, responds only to painful stimuli
- ▼ Glasgow coma scale calculated at 7:
  - ▼ eye opening, none (1)
  - ▼ verbal response, none (1)
  - ▼ motor response, localizes (5)

SENSORY EXAM

- ▼ localizes painful stimuli and moves all extremities except in left femur

BACK

▼ no deformity
▼ no discoloration
▼ no trauma noted

Scenario Progression and Analysis: This scenario is a trauma scenario, with the one twist that the patient is also suffering from a narcotic overdose. EMT-As and Is should be tested on how quickly they diagnose the problems, treat the injuries, package the patient and transport, or call for an ALS unit. For the paramedics, the patient's level of consciousness will improve slightly if naloxone is given at any time in this scenario, with vital signs remaining the same. If this is not addressed or BTLS/PHTLS guidelines are not followed, then the patient should deteriorate.

SUGGESTED TREATMENT

EMT-A Level

▼ Conduct Scene Survey with patient removal, as per local protocols.
▼ Conduct Primary Assessment, while extinguishing any smoldering or active burning.
  ▼ Remove all clothing and jewelry.
▼ Airway management should include proper application of the bag-valve-mask device with 100% O_2 administration.
  ▼ Position patient properly.
  ▼ Open airway with modified jaw thrust method.
  ▼ Insert naso/oropharyngeal airway.
▼ Maintain cervical spine manually during and after airway management.
▼ Secure patient with cervical immobilization devices and backboard.
▼ Conduct MAST survey.
▼ Apply sterile burn sheets to burn areas.
▼ Apply pneumatic antishock garment.
▼ Reassess airway, breathing, circulation, and level of consciousness.
▼ Apply blanket to prevent further heat loss.
▼ Transport ASAP or call for an ALS unit.
▼ Conduct Secondary Assessment
▼ Splint femur fracture, as per local protocols.
▼ Notify appropriate receiving facility.

EMT-I Level

▼ Treatment is the same as above, but includes the following:
▼ Airway management should include insertion of an esophageal airway.

- ▼ Place in sniffing position.
- ▼ Assess lung sounds.
- ▼ Establish at least two large-bore IVs, infusing either normal saline or Ringer's lactate, open.
  - ▼ Select sites other than burned areas.
- ▼ Reassess airway, breathing, circulation, and level of consciousness.
- ▼ Apply automatic external defibrillator, as per local protocols.

EMT-P Level:

- ▼ Conduct Scene Survey with patient removal, as per local protocols.
- ▼ Conduct Primary Assessment, while extinguishing any smoldering or active burning.
  - ▼ Rapidly assess ECG rhythm, showing a sinus tachycardia.
  - ▼ Remove all clothing and jewelry.
- ▼ Airway management should include proper application of the bag-valve-mask device with 100% O_2 administration.
  - ▼ Position patient properly.
  - ▼ Open airway with modified jaw thrust method.
  - ▼ Insert naso/oropharyngeal airway.
- ▼ Complete oral intubation with appropriate-sized tube.
  - ▼ Hyperventilate before and after.
  - ▼ No longer than 30 seconds.
  - ▼ Assess lung sounds.
- ▼ Maintain cervical spine manually, during and after airway management.
- ▼ Secure patient with cervical immobilization devices and backboard.
- ▼ Conduct MAST survey.
- ▼ Apply pneumatic antishock garment.
- ▼ Apply sterile burn sheets to burn areas.
- ▼ Reassess airway, breathing, circulation, and level of consciousness.
- ▼ Apply blanket to prevent further heat loss.
- ▼ Administer 2 mg of naloxone, ET, and titrate to respirations.
- ▼ (New ACLS guidelines suggest a 2 to 2.5 times increase of medication dosage if given ET for proper absorbtion.)
- ▼ Reassess airway, breathing, circulation, and level of consciousness.

AT THIS TIME, THE PATIENT'S LEVEL OF CONSCIOUSNESS INCREASES TO BEING SOME-WHAT RESPONSIVE TO VERBAL STIMULI.

- ▼ Transport ASAP.
- ▼ Consider aerosol treatment, as per local protocols.
- ▼ Establish two large-bore IVs, infusing Ringer's lactate or normal saline, open.
  - ▼ Select sites other than burned areas.

- Reassess airway, breathing, circulation, and level of consciousness.
- Conduct Secondary Assessment.
- Splint femur fracture, as per local protocols.
- Notify appropriate receiving facility.

ADDITIONAL PROBLEMS

Depending on the level of the candidate, the following problems can be added to the scenario:

1. The patient's level of consciousness can rapidly increase and he can become extremely combative after the naloxone administration.
2. The patient can extubate himself with airway compromise.
3. IV access can be limited because of the burn injuries and require external jugular insertion.
4. Additional problem of infectious diseases can be added because of the IV drug abuse history.
5. Associated injuries can cause neurovascular compromise.
6. The additional problem of cervicalspine injury with neurogenic shock may be added to the scenario.
7. Airway burn injuries can become more severe and cause respiratory arrest.
8. Any location can be given to test the candidate's street or address competency, using local running cards.
9. Any scene hazard can be incorporated at the presenter's discretion. (This is in addition to or replacement of those already mentioned.)
10. After IV lines have been established, the patient can deteriorate and go into cardiac arrest to further test the candidate's knowledge.

SUMMARY

This patient suffers from heroine overdose, as well as being a trauma victim with respiratory compromise due to an explosion and fire, prior to your arrival. In any situation like this, naloxone should be considered due to the level of consciousness and possible drug history. Proper treatment of the burns would include prevention of further contamination, early airway management, and vigorous fluid resuscitation, as well as management of hypothermia. This patient also has a broken femur and an unstable pelvis, and these would be treated by initial splinting with the antishock garment and then, later, for the femur, with a traction device. Because of the potential toxic gas and burn injury associated with inhalation during a fire, early intubation and respiratory support with 100% oxygen should be performed. The treatment of bronchial spasm should be as local protocols dictate, but considered. Rapid transport to the appropriate medical facility is another key to this scenario.

It is important to note that the incidence of heroine abuse seems to be increasing in some areas.

TRAUMA SCENARIO 4

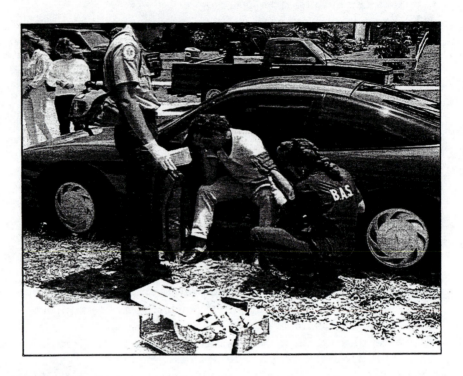

Type: Trauma.
Scenario moulage/prop list: Live model or mannequin sitting in passenger car, old shirt with moulage blood around a puncture hole, grease paint for jugular disten- tion and pale skin color, medical alert bracelet, glycerin water in spray bottle for skin, bullet hole moulaged with mortician's wax (street setting with motor vehicle).

INITIAL SCENE DESCRIPTION

Dispatch Information

LOCATION: City street, urban area
NUMBER OF VICTIMS: 1, possibly more
TYPE OF SITUATION: Shooting
HAZARDS: Police on scene, scene secure
WEATHER CONDITIONS: Clear, hot night
TIME OF DAY: 0200 hours

Scene

Dispatch informs you of a possible shooting in the downtown area. The scene is an urban street. Police have secured the area and you arrive to find a 22-year-old male seated in the driver's seat of a passenger car. He is crying loudly from abdominal pain. You note a small, blood-soaked hole in the left, upper quadrant of the abdominal portion of his shirt, with minimal external bleeding.

The police notify you that the patient said he was driving, when suddenly he heard a loud noise and felt a sharp pain in his abdomen. The officer states that, because of the neighborhood, "this may have been a drug buy gone sour", You observe that there are no bullet holes in the vehicle and that the window is down and intact.

PRIMARY ASSESSMENT FINDINGS

SCENE SURVEY

- ▼ urban street with police present
- ▼ crowd forming
- ▼ only one victim found

AIRWAY/CERVICAL SPINE

- ▼ airway open
- ▼ no complaint of neck pain
- ▼ signs of trauma
- ▼ neck veins distended

BREATHING

- ▼ 28 breaths per minute, shallow
- ▼ chest rise decreased on the left
- ▼ lungs clear right side, diminished left side
- ▼ percussion reveals hyperresonance to left chest

CIRCULATION/HEMORRHAGE CONTROL

- ▼ rapid, weak carotid pulse at 120
- ▼ rapid, weak radial pulse at 120
- ▼ capillary refill delayed to 5 seconds
- ▼ small amount of blood soaked around hole in front of shirt
- ▼ no other external bleeding observed

DISABILITY

- ▼ (A, V, P, U) alert, rapidly deteriorating

EXPOSE AND EXAMINE

- ▼ bullet wound in left, upper abdominal quadrant
- ▼ medic alert bracelet: "seizures"

- ▼ skin turgor good
- ▼ skin color pale
- ▼ skin cool and diaphoretic to touch
- ▼ weight estimated at 160 lb

SECONDARY ASSESSMENT FINDINGS

VITAL SIGNS

- ▼ respirations, 28 and shallow
- ▼ pulse, 120
- ▼ blood pressure, 90/40
- ▼ ECG, a sinus tachycardia

HISTORY

- ▼ as above, except for the following:
    - ▼ A   none
    - ▼ M   phenobarbital, depakene
    - ▼ P   seizure disorder
    - ▼ L   couple of beers 1 hour ago, no food
    - ▼ E   as above, per patient

HEAD

- ▼ no visible trauma
- ▼ no deformity on palpation
- ▼ pupils equal and reactive to light

NECK

- ▼ trachea midline
- ▼ neck veins distended
- ▼ no deformity
- ▼ no discoloration

CHEST

- ▼ no visible deformity
- ▼ no discoloration
- ▼ unequal chest wall movement on the left
- ▼ lung sounds clear right side, diminished left
- ▼ percussion reveals hyperresonance to left side of chest
- ▼ no deformity, tenderness, or crepitus on palpation

ABDOMEN

- small-caliber bullet hole upper left
- abdomen distended
- rigid and tender to palpation
- (if checked, bowel sounds absent)
- pelvic rock stable

EXTREMITIES

- no deformity
- no discoloration
- no visible signs of trauma
- capillary refill delayed to 5 seconds
- medic alert bracelet on right wrist
- weak, rapid distal pulses palpated
- skin turgor good
- skin color pale
- skin cool and diaphoretic to touch
- no tenderness, crepitus, or swelling
- movement of all extremities equal

NEUROLOGICAL

- conscious and alert, but deteriorating
- Glascow coma scale calculated at 15:
  - eye opening, spontaneous (4)
  - verbal response is oriented (5)
  - motor response, obeys (6)

SENSORY EXAM

- no deficit in sensory or motor function

BACK

- no deformity
- no discoloration
- no trauma noted

Scenario Progression and Analysis: The patient's respirations become increasingly more labored while the rate increases. The level of consciousness continues to decrease to unresponsiveness. The blood pressure should begin to drop rapidly. The EMT-As and Is should be tested on how quickly they diagnose the problem, initiate treatment, and transport and/or call for an ALS Unit. For the paramedics, if the pneumothorax is noted early and treated correctly, the patient should remain the same. If the hypotension is aggressively managed, the vital signs will only fall slowly. If BTLS/PHTLS guidelines are not followed or the pneumothorax is not treated, the patient should go into cardiac arrest.

SUGGESTED TREATMENT

EMT-A Level

▼ Conduct Scene Survey.
▼ Conduct Primary Assessment.
▼ Airway management should include high-flow O_2 administration with a mask.
▼ Maintain cervical spine manually during and after airway management.
▼ Secure patient with cervical immobilization to backboard.
▼ Conduct MAST survey.
▼ Apply pneumatic antishock garment, as per local protocols.
▼ Reassess airway, breathing, circulation, and level of consciousness.

AT THIS TIME, THE PATIENT BECOMES UNRESPONSIVE (WITH A PULSE OF 140 BPM AND RESPIRATIONS OF 44).

▼ Airway management should include proper application of the bag-valve-mask device with 100% O_2 administration.
  ▼ Position patient properly.
  ▼ Open airway with head-tilt, chin lift.
  ▼ Insert naso/oropharyngeal airway.
▼ Transport ASAP or call for an ALS Unit, as per local protocols.
▼ Conduct Secondary Assessment.
▼ Dress wound.
▼ Notify appropriate receiving facility.

EMT-I Level

▼ Treatment is the same as above, but includes the following:
▼ Airway management should include insertion of an esophageal airway.
  ▼ Place in sniffing position.
  ▼ Assess lung sounds.
▼ Establish at least two large-bore IVs, infusing either Ringer's lactate or normal saline, open.
▼ Reassess airway, breathing, circulation, and level of consciousness.
▼ Apply automatic external defibrillator, as per local protocols.

EMT-P Level

▾ Conduct Scene Survey.

▾ Conduct Primary Assessment with rapid assessment of ECG, showing a sinus tachycardia.

▾ Airway management should include high-flow O_2 administration with a mask.

▾ Maintain cervical spine immobilization during and after airway management. (Some may choose to decompress the chest at this time.)

▾ Secure patient with cervical immobilization devices to backboard.

▾ Conduct MAST survey.

▾ Apply pneumatic antishock garment, as per local protocols.

▾ Reassess ECG, airway, breathing, circulation, and level of consciousness.

AT THIS TIME, THE PATIENT BECOMES UNRESPONSIVE (WITH A PULSE OF 140 BPM, RESPIRATIONS OF 44, AND TOTAL ABSENCE OF BREATH SOUNDS ON LEFT SIDE).

▾ Airway management should include proper application of the bag-valve-mask device with 100% O_2 administration.

  ▾ Position patient properly.
  ▾ Open airway with head-tilt, chin-lift.
  ▾ Insert naso/oropharyngeal airway.

▾ Decompress left side of chest, as per local protocols.

▾ Reassess ECG, airway, breathing, circulation, and level of consciousness.

AT THIS TIME, THE PATIENT REMAINS UNRESPONSIVE (BUT RESPIRATIONS SLOW TO 28 BPM, WHILE THE PULSEINCREASES TO 144).

▾ Complete oral intubation with appropriate-sized tube.

  ▾ Hyperventilate before and after.
  ▾ No longer than 30 seconds.
  ▾ Reassess lung sounds.

▾ Transport ASAP.

▾ Establish at least two large-bore IVs, infusing either normal saline or Ringer's lactate, open.

▾ Reassess ECG, airway, breathing, circulation, and level of consciousness.

▾ Conduct Secondary Assessment.

▾ Dress wound.

▾ Notify appropriate receiving facility.

ADDITIONAL PROBLEMS

Depending on the level of the candidate, the following problems can be added to the scenario:

1. The bystanders can become violent during the course of the scenario and force the team to remove the patient more quickly or block their evacuation.
2. The patient's transport can be delayed for any reason, requiring treatment be done on scene.
3. During airway management, the endotracheal tube placement can take too long or be imporperly placed in the esophagus, requiring that the candidate should use an esophageal airway.
4. Seizure activity can occur as the blood pressure decreases.
5. A narcotic drug abuse or diabetic history can be included requiring that the candidate address these problems with naloxone and 50% dextrose.
6. After IV lines have been established, the patient can deteriorate and go into cardiac arrest to further test the candidates knowledge.
7. Any location can be given to test the candidate's street or address competency, using local running cards.
8. Any scene hazard can be incorporated, at the presenter's discretion. (This is in addition to or replacement of those already mentioned).

SUMMARY

This is a typical trauma scenario. The bullet struck this patient's left kidney and then lodged in his left lung, causing a pneumothorax and an internal bleed. The treatment is directed toward assessment and treatment of life-threatening injuries and rapid transport to the appropriate receiving facility. No delay in transport should occur. Scene safety should be the first priority in this scenario because of the violent nature of the call.

Because of the present controversy concerning the application of the pneumatic antishock trousers in cases of penetrating injuries of the chest and abdomen, local protocols must dictate their use in scenarios like this. The authors chose to use the antishock trousers in the suggested treatment portion, since they are still widely utilized throughout EMS. When more conclusive information is available as to the effectiveness and indications for the use of this device, then areas like this may seem no longer debatable. You are encouraged to modify the treatment according to the mainstream of information available.

BIBLIOGRAPHY

American Academy of Pediatrics, Pediatric Advanced Life Support, Dallas, Texas American Heart Association, 1988.

ANTHONY, C., and G. THIBODEAU, *Structure and Function of the Body*, 6th ed. St. Louis, Mo.: C.V. Mosby Co., 1980.

BARSAN, W.G., and others, "Blood Levels of Diazepam After Endotracheal Administration in Dogs", *Emerg. Med.* (November 1982) 11:242–247.

BLEDSOE, BRYAN E., and others, *Paramedic Emergency Care*: Englewood Cliffs, N.J.: Prentice Hall, 1991.

CAMPBELL, JOHN EMORY, *Basic Trauma Life Support*, 2nd ed. Englewood Cliffs, N.J.: Prentice Hall, 1988.

CAROLINE, NANCY L., *Emergency Care in the Streets*, 3rd ed. Boston: Little, Brown and Co., 1987.

CHUNG, EDWARD K., *Cardiac Emergency Care*, Malverne, Pa.: Lea and Febiger, 1991.

Department of Transportation, *Prehospital Environment, Roles and Responsibilities*, Washington, D.C.: Department of Transportation, 1985.

Emergency Cardiac Care Committee and Subcommittees, American Heart Association. Guidelines for Cardiopulmonary Resuscitation and Emergency Cardiac Care, *JAMA* 1992; 268 (16) 2171–2298.

GOODMAN, LOUIS S., and A. G. GILLMAN, *The Pharmacological Basis of Therapeutics*, 7th ed. New York: Macmillan, Inc., 1985.

HAFEN, BRENT Q., and KEITH J. KARREN, *Prehospital Emergency Care*, 3rd ed. Englewood, Colo.: Morton Publishing Co., 1989.

Prehospital Trauma Life Support, 2nd ed. Akron, Ohio: Emergency Training, 1990.

ROSEN, PETER, and others, *Emergency Medicine, Concepts and Clinical Practice*, 2nd ed. St. Louis, Mo.: The C. V. Mosby Co., 1988.

STEILL, I.G., HERBERT, P.C., Wietzman, B.N. and others, *"High-Dose Epinephrine in Adult*

Cardiac Arrest", N. Eng. J. Med., 327, 1992, pp. 1045–50.

SULLIVAN, TIMOTHY J., "Cross-reactions among Furosemide, Hydrochlorothiazide, and Sulfonamides," *JAMA,* (January 1991), 265(1):120–121.

THADEPALLI, HARAGOPAL, *Infectious Diseases.* Garden City, New York: Medical Examination Publishing Co., 1980.

TORNHEIM, PATRICIA A., *"Effect of Furosemide on Experimental Traumatic Cerebral Edema,"* Neurosurgery, (January 1979), 4(1):48–52.

WILLARD, J.E., LANGE, R.A, and HILLIS, L.D., *"The Use of Aspirin in Ischemic Heart Disease,"* N. Eng. J. Med., 327 1992, 175–81.

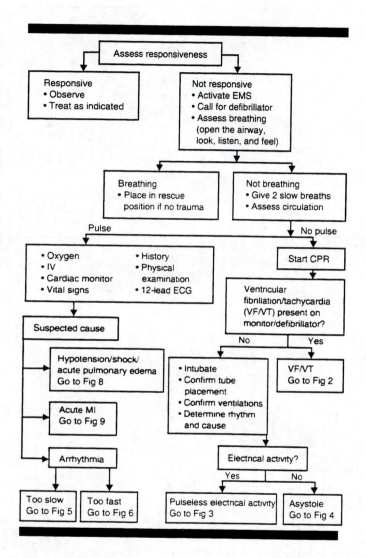

Figure 1—Universal algorithm for adult emergency cardiac care (ECC).
Reproduced with permission. Guidelines for Cardiopulmonary Resuscitation and Emergency Cardiac Care, 1992. Copyright American Heart Association.

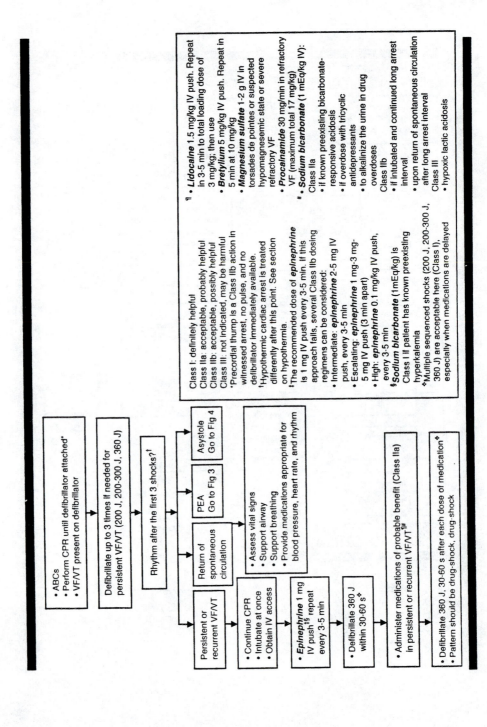

Figure 2—Algorithm for ventricular fibrillation and pulseless ventricular tachycardia (VF/VT). Reproduced with permission. Guidelines for Cardiopulmonary Resuscitation and Emergency Cardiac Care, 1992. Copyright American Heart Association.

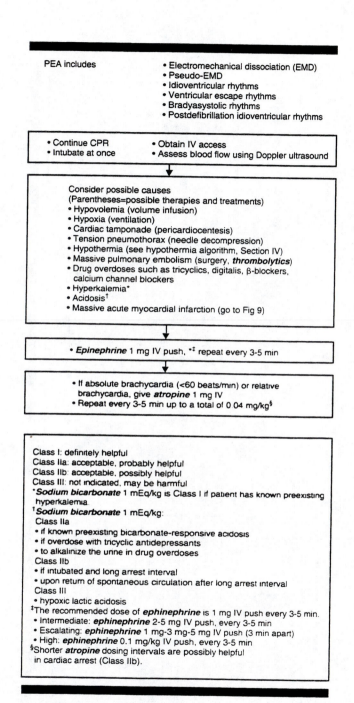

PEA includes
- Electromechanical dissociation (EMD)
- Pseudo-EMD
- Idioventricular rhythms
- Ventricular escape rhythms
- Bradyasystolic rhythms
- Postdefibrillation idioventricular rhythms

- Continue CPR
- Intubate at once
- Obtain IV access
- Assess blood flow using Doppler ultrasound

↓

Consider possible causes
(Parentheses=possible therapies and treatments)
- Hypovolemia (volume infusion)
- Hypoxia (ventilation)
- Cardiac tamponade (pericardiocentesis)
- Tension pneumothorax (needle decompression)
- Hypothermia (see hypothermia algorithm, Section IV)
- Massive pulmonary embolism (surgery, **thrombolytics**)
- Drug overdoses such as tricyclics, digitalis, β-blockers, calcium channel blockers
- Hyperkalemia*
- Acidosis†
- Massive acute myocardial infarction (go to Fig 9)

↓

- **Epinephrine** 1 mg IV push, *‡ repeat every 3-5 min

↓

- If absolute brachycardia (<60 beats/min) or relative brachycardia, give **atropine** 1 mg IV
- Repeat every 3-5 min up to a total of 0 04 mg/kg§

Class I: definitely helpful
Class IIa: acceptable, probably helpful
Class IIb: acceptable, possibly helpful
Class III: not indicated, may be harmful
*Sodium bicarbonate 1 mEq/kg is Class I if patient has known preexisting hyperkalemia.
†Sodium bicarbonate 1 mEq/kg:
Class IIa
- if known preexisting bicarbonate-responsive acidosis
- if overdose with tricyclic antidepressants
- to alkalinize the urine in drug overdoses
Class IIb
- if intubated and long arrest interval
- upon return of spontaneous circulation after long arrest interval
Class III
- hypoxic lactic acidosis
‡The recommended dose of **ephinephrine** is 1 mg IV push every 3-5 min.
- Intermediate: **ephinephrine** 2-5 mg IV push, every 3-5 min
- Escalating: **ephinephrine** 1 mg-3 mg-5 mg IV push (3 min apart)
- High: **ephinephrine** 0.1 mg/kg IV push, every 3-5 min
§Shorter **atropine** dosing intervals are possibly helpful in cardiac arrest (Class IIb).

Figure 3—Algorithm for pulseless electrical activity (PEA) (electromechanical dissociation {EMD}).
Reproduced with permission. Guidelines for Cardiopulmonary Resuscitation and Emergency Cardiac Care, 1992. Copyright American Heart Association.

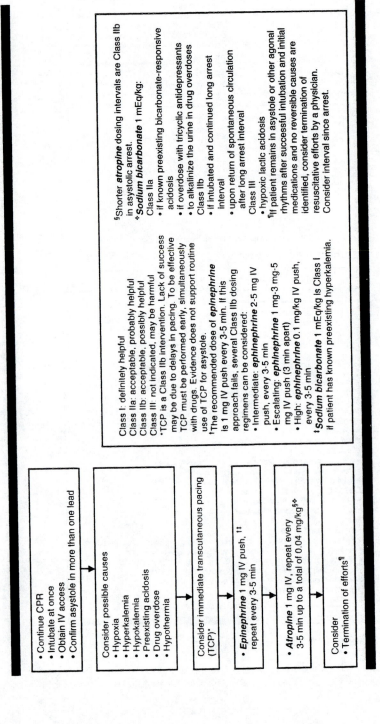

- Continue CPR
- Intubate at once
- Obtain IV access
- Confirm asystole in more than one lead

↓

Consider possible causes
- Hypoxia
- Hyperkalemia
- Hypokalemia
- Preexisting acidosis
- Drug overdose
- Hypothermia

↓

Consider immediate transcutaneous pacing (TCP)*

↓

- *Epinephrine* 1 mg IV push,†‡ repeat every 3-5 min

↓

- *Atropine* 1 mg IV, repeat every 3-5 min up to a total of 0.04 mg/kg§✦

↓

Consider
- Termination of efforts¶

Class I: definitely helpful
Class IIa: acceptable, probably helpful
Class IIb: acceptable, possibly helpful
Class III: not indicated, may be harmful
*TCP is a Class IIb intervention. Lack of success may be due to delays in pacing. To be effective TCP must be performed early, simultaneously with drugs. Evidence does not support routine use of TCP for asystole.
†The recommended dose of *epinephrine* is 1 mg IV push every 3-5 min. If this approach fails, several Class IIb dosing regimens can be considered:
- Intermediate: *epinephrine* 2-5 mg IV push, every 3-5 min
- Escalating: *epinephrine* 1 mg-3 mg-5 mg IV push (3 min apart)
- High: *epinephrine* 0.1 mg/kg IV push, every 3-5 min
‡*Sodium bicarbonate* 1 mEq/kg is Class I if patient has known preexisting hyperkalemia.

§Shorter *atropine* dosing intervals are Class IIb in asystolic arrest.
✦*Sodium bicarbonate* 1 mEq/kg:
Class IIa
- if known preexisting bicarbonate-responsive acidosis
- if overdose with tricyclic antidepressants
- to alkalinize the urine in drug overdoses
Class IIb
- if intubated and continued long arrest interval
- upon return of spontaneous circulation after long arrest interval
Class III
- hypoxic lactic acidosis
¶If patient remains in asystole or other agonal rhythms after successful intubation and initial medications and no reversible causes are identified, consider termination of resuscitative efforts by a physician. Consider interval since arrest.

Figure 4—Asytole treatment algorithm.
Reproduced with permission. Guidelines for Cardiopulmonary Resuscitation and Emergency Cardiac Car, 1992. Copyright American Heart Association.

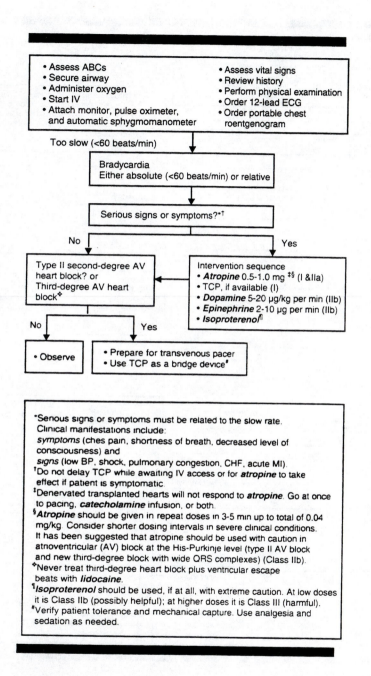

- Assess ABCs
- Secure airway
- Administer oxygen
- Start IV
- Attach monitor, pulse oximeter, and automatic sphygmomanometer

- Assess vital signs
- Review history
- Perform physical examination
- Order 12-lead ECG
- Order portable chest roentgenogram

Too slow (<60 beats/min)

Bradycardia
Either absolute (<60 beats/min) or relative

Serious signs or symptoms?*†

No

Type II second-degree AV heart block? or
Third-degree AV heart block✣

Yes

Intervention sequence
- *Atropine* 0.5-1.0 mg ‡§ (I &IIa)
- TCP, if available (I)
- *Dopamine* 5-20 µg/kg per min (IIb)
- *Epinephrine* 2-10 µg per min (IIb)
- *Isoproterenol*‖

No

- Observe

Yes

- Prepare for transvenous pacer
- Use TCP as a bridge device＊

*Serious signs or symptoms must be related to the slow rate.
Clinical manifestations include:
symptoms (ches pain, shortness of breath, decreased level of consciousness) and
signs (low BP, shock, pulmonary congestion, CHF, acute MI).
†Do not delay TCP while awaiting IV access or for *atropine* to take effect if patient is symptomatic.
‡Denervated transplanted hearts will not respond to *atropine*. Go at once to pacing, *catecholamine* infusion, or both.
§*Atropine* should be given in repeat doses in 3-5 min up to total of 0.04 mg/kg. Consider shorter dosing intervals in severe clinical conditions. It has been suggested that atropine should be used with caution in atrioventricular (AV) block at the His-Purkinje level (type II AV block and new third-degree block with wide QRS complexes) (Class IIb).
✣Never treat third-degree heart block plus ventricular escape beats with *lidocaine*.
‖*Isoproterenol* should be used, if at all, with extreme caution. At low doses it is Class IIb (possibly helpful); at higher doses it is Class III (harmful).
＊Verify patient tolerance and mechanical capture. Use analgesia and sedation as needed.

Figure 5—Bradycardia algorithm (with the patient not in cardiac arrest). Reproduced with permission. Guidelines for Cardiopulmonary Resuscitation and Emergency Cardiac Care, 1992. Copyright American Heart Association.

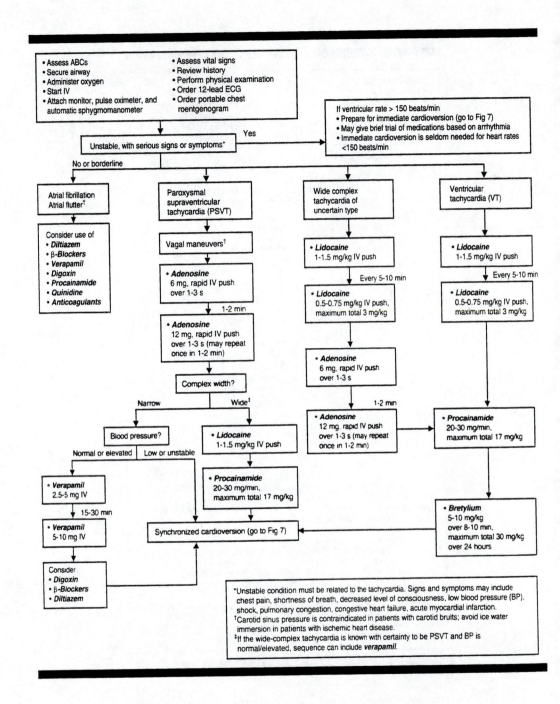

Figure 6—Tachycardia algorithm.
Reproduced with permission. Guidelines for Cardiopulmonary Resuscitation and Emergency Cardiac Care, 1992. Copyright American Heart Association.

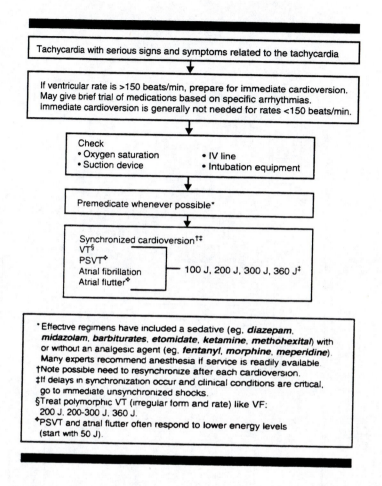

Tachycardia with serious signs and symptoms related to the tachycardia

If ventricular rate is >150 beats/min, prepare for immediate cardioversion.
May give brief trial of medications based on specific arrhythmias.
Immediate cardioversion is generally not needed for rates <150 beats/min.

Check
• Oxygen saturation
• Suction device
• IV line
• Intubation equipment

Premedicate whenever possible*

Synchronized cardioversion†‡
VT$
PSVT✦
Atrial fibrillation
Atrial flutter✦   100 J, 200 J, 300 J, 360 J‡

* Effective regimens have included a sedative (eg, *diazepam*,
  midazolam, *barbiturates*, *etomidate*, *ketamine*, *methohexital*) with
  or without an analgesic agent (eg, *fentanyl*, *morphine*, *meperidine*).
  Many experts recommend anesthesia if service is readily available.
†Note possible need to resynchronize after each cardioversion.
‡If delays in synchronization occur and clinical conditions are critical,
  go to immediate unsynchronized shocks.
§Treat polymorphic VT (irregular form and rate) like VF:
  200 J, 200-300 J, 360 J.
✦PSVT and atrial flutter often respond to lower energy levels
  (start with 50 J).

Figure 7—Electrical cardioversion algorithm (with the patient not in car-
diac arrest).
Reproduced with permission. Guidelines for Cardiopulmonary
Resuscitation and Emergency Cardiac Care, 1992. Copyright American
Heart Association.

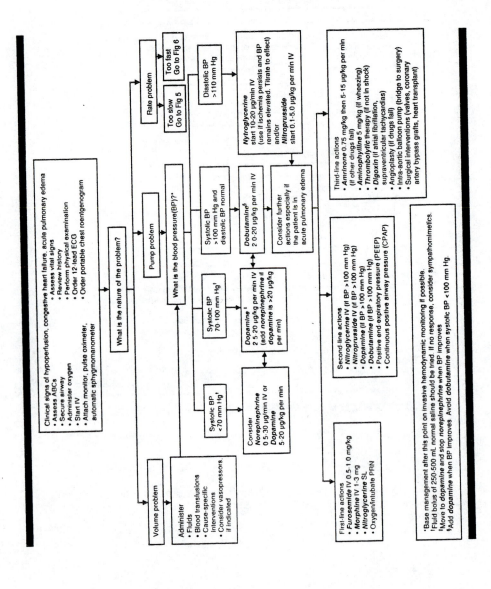

Clinical signs of hypoperfusion, congestive heart failure, acute pulmonary edema
- Assess ABCs
- Secure airway
- Administer oxygen
- Start IV
- Attach monitor, pulse oximeter, automatic sphygmomanometer
- Assess vital signs
- Review history
- Perform physical examination
- Order 12-lead ECG
- Order portable chest roentgenogram

What is the nature of the problem?

Volume problem

Administer
- Fluids
- Blood transfusions
- Cause-specific interventions
- Consider vasopressors, if indicated

Pump problem

Rate problem

Too slow
Go to Fig 5

Too fast
Go to Fig 6

What is the blood pressure(BP)?

Systolic BP
<70 mm Hg‖

Consider
Norepinephrine
0.5-30 µg/min IV or
Dopamine
5-20 µg/kg per min

Systolic BP
70-100 mm Hg‖

Dopamine ‖
2.5-20 µg/kg per min IV
(add *norepinephrine* if
dopamine is >20 µg/kg
per min)

Systolic BP
>100 mm Hg and
diastolic BP normal

Dobutamine §
2.0-20 µg/kg per min IV

Diastolic BP
>110 mm Hg

Nytroglycerine
start 10-20 µg/min IV
(use if ischemia persists and BP
remains elevated. Titrate to effect)
and/or
Nitroprusside
start 0.1-5.0 µg/kg per min IV

Consider further
actions especially if
the patient is in
acute pulmonary edema

First-line actions
- *Furosemide* IV 0.5-1.0 mg/kg
- *Morphine* IV 1-3 mg
- *Nitroglycerine* SL
- Oxygen/intubate PRN

Second line actions
- *Nitroglycerine IV* (if BP >100 mm Hg)
- *Nitroprusside IV* (if BP >100 mm Hg)
- *Dopamine* (if BP >100 mm Hg)
- *Dobutamine* (if BP >100 mm Hg)
- Positive end expiratory pressure (PEEP)
- Continuous positive airway pressure (CPAP)

Third-line actions
- *Amrinone* 0.75 mg/kg then 5-15 µg/kg per min
  (if other drugs fail)
- *Aminophylline* 5 mg/kg (if wheezing)
- *Thrombolytic* therapy (if not in shock)
- *Digoxin* (if atrial fibrillation,
  supraventricular tachycardias)
- Angioplasty (if drugs fail)
- Intra-aortic balloon pump (bridge to surgery)
- Surgical interventions (valves, coronary
  artery bypass grafts, heart transplant)

• Base management after this point on invasive hemodynamic monitoring if possible.
‖ Fluid bolus of 250-500 mL normal saline should be tried. If no response, consider sympathomimetics.
• Move to *dopamine* and stop *norepinephrine* when BP improves. Avoid *dobutamine* when systolic BP <100 mm Hg.
§ Add *dopamine* when BP improves.

Figure 8—Algorithm for hypotension, shock, and acute pulmonary edema.
Reproduced with permission. Guidelines for Cardiopulmonary Resuscitation and Emergency
Cardiac Care, 1992. Copyright American Heart Association.